Family Work
for Schizophrenia

Family Work for Schizophrenia

Second edition

Elizabeth Kuipers

Julian Leff

and Dominic Lam

Gaskell

© The Royal College of Psychiatrists 2002, 2006
First edition © The Royal College of Psychiatrists 1992

First published 1992
This edition published 2002
Reprinted 2005, revised format 2006

Gaskell is an imprint of the Royal College of Psychiatrists, 17 Belgrave Square, London SW1X 8PG
http://www.rcpsych.ac.uk

British Library Cataloguing-in-Publication Data.
A catalogue record for this book is available from the British Library.
ISBN 1-901242-77-3

Distributed in North America by Balogh International Inc.

The views presented in this book do not necessarily reflect those of the Royal College of
Psychiatrists, and the publishers are not responsible for any error of omission or fact.

The Royal College of Psychiatrists is a registered charity (no. 228636).

Printed in Great Britain by Bell & Bain Limited, Glasgow.

"Don't turn your back"

Don't turn your back on my brother
Just because he does not fit
into your world.
His torment is real
and he would change it if he could.

His illness is not something
you can see
but is real, all too real,
nonetheless,
and the boy we know is lost to us.
Like a missing child
the pain never dies
but haunts us with hopes
that some day
we will find him again.

An excerpt from a poem by Barbara Bingham. Reprinted with the author's permission from the *World Schizophrenia Fellowship Newsletter,* September 1991.

The authors

Elizabeth Kuipers is Professor of Clinical Psychology at the Institute of Psychiatry, King's College London, and Honorary Consultant Clinical Psychologist, South London and Maudsley Trust.

Julian Leff is Head of the Section of Social Psychiatry and Professor of Social and Cultural Psychiatry at the Institute of Psychiatry, King's College London, and Honorary Consultant Psychiatrist, South London and Maudsley Trust.

Dominic Lam is Senior Lecturer in Clinical Psychology at the Institute of Psychiatry, King's College London, and Honorary Consultant Clinical Psychologist, South London and Maudsley Trust.

Contents

Acknowledgements

We would like to thank all the families we have met and talked with over the years, for their contribution, insights and humour even in the most difficult situations. We learned a lot from them about coping with problems, and came to appreciate their ingenuity and creativity.

We are very grateful to the 20 psychiatric nurses who completed our first two training courses in family work for schizophrenia. They taught us a great deal about how to teach. Dr Peter Burnett and Mrs Ellen Wheeler joined our discussions throughout the writing of the first edition of this book and made many valuable contributions from the viewpoints of a family therapist and a carer, respectively. We wish to acknowledge with gratitude the major role played by Dr Ruth Berkowitz in developing and shaping our form of family work during the many years she was a member of our team. An excellent standard of typing by Mrs Yvonne Waters smoothed the production of the manuscript.

Part I

Introduction

CHAPTER 1

Introduction to our approach

From the late 1960s to early 1970s, researchers at the Medical Research Council's Social Psychiatry Unit in London were investigating whether family atmosphere can influence the course of illness in schizophrenia. They found that patients living with a critical or overinvolved relative were more prone to relapse. They coined the term 'high expressed emotion' to describe such families (Brown & Rutter, 1966; Brown et al, 1972). These findings were first replicated in the Medical Research Council's Unit, with a shorter interview schedule, by Vaughn & Leff (1976). Since then further replications have been reported throughout the world and in different cultures (Vaughn et al, 1984; Jenkins et al, 1986; Leff et al, 1987; Mino et al, 1990). More recently, however, a few studies failed to replicate the earlier findings. Parker & Hadzi-Pavlovic (1990) summarised the recent controversial studies. None the less, an aggregate analysis of 25 studies, by Bebbington & Kuipers (1994), confirmed the association between relatives' expressed emotion (EE) and the course of schizophrenia. The predictive value of EE has also been confirmed more recently by a meta-analysis of published studies (Butzlaff & Hooley, 1999).

Expressed emotion is essentially a clinical concept. It contributes little to our understanding of the aetiology of schizophrenia, but is a robust predictor of its course when someone with the illness lives with relatives. The model of treatment described in this manual stems from this predictive power of EE.

Research on EE has been extended to professional carers, who have been found sometimes to develop critical attitudes towards patients with schizophrenia which are comparable to those expressed by some family members (Ball et al, 1992; Moore & Kuipers, 1992; Snyder et al, 1992; Willetts & Leff, 1997). In the most recent study, Willetts & Leff found that professional staff who were critical towards one patient in their care were always non-critical towards another. This important observation demonstrates that EE is an interactional measure and does not represent an emotional attitude which pervades all the person's relationships. Hence a change in attitude is always a possibility.

Another direction in which EE research has developed is in extending the range of diagnoses in which it has been investigated. These include manic–depressive illness (Miklowitz et al, 1983), depressive neurosis (Hooley et al, 1986; Okasha et al, 1994), post-traumatic stress disorder (Tarrier et al, 1999) and eating disorders (Fischmann-Havstad & Marston, 1984). Non-psychiatric conditions studied include diabetes (Sensky et al, 1991; Koenigsberg et al, 1993), epilepsy, Parkinson's disease (MacCarthy et al, 1989) and inflammatory bowel disease (Vaughn et al, 1999). In each of these conditions, relatives have been found to express high EE. This informs us that such attitudes are not specifically linked to schizophrenia and therefore cannot be a prime cause of this condition, a reassuring message to give to relatives. It appears that high EE can develop in response to any long-term or recurrent condition, whether it is psychiatric or non-psychiatric in nature.

What are the emotions measured by EE?

The measurement of EE is a research technique and the components of the EE index – critical comments, hostility and overinvolvement – are technical terms and not the names of emotions. However, clearly recognisable emotions give rise to the responses and behaviour that EE measures. Criticism is a direct expression of anger, and the number of critical comments made during an interview indicates how angry the carer is with the patient. Hostility is an extreme form of criticism and represents a high intensity of anger, which may be accompanied by rejection of the patient.

Overinvolvement is fuelled by a mixture of anxiety and guilt. Guilt stems from feeling responsible for the patient's illness, and is much more common among parents than other relatives or professional carers. The sense of guilt may impel relatives to try to do everything possible for patients, to make up for the impact of the illness on their life. Unfortunately, this results in patients becoming increasingly dependent on their relative and anxious about their ability to cope on their own. Hence both partners in an overinvolved relationship are made very anxious by the prospect of separation.

Low-EE relatives and the importance of warmth

The term 'high EE' is somewhat misleading. It is often interpreted to mean that it is preferable for family members to suppress all emotions in the presence of the patient. Nothing could be further from the truth. There is strong evidence that the negative emotions of criticism, hostility and overinvolvement tend to worsen the outcome for people with schizophrenia and should be avoided if possible. But high levels of warmth improve the course of the condition, and one of the aims of family work is to increase the expression of warmth by relatives. To avoid misunderstanding, it would have been preferable to label the measure 'high negative EE', but the term coined by its originators, George Brown and Michael Rutter, is too well established to be changed now.

Low-EE relatives are not simply neutral

It is incorrect to think of low-EE relatives as being characterised only by a lack of criticism, hostility and overinvolvement. Rather they possess a range of positive coping strategies which they have worked out for themselves. They differ fundamentally from high-EE relatives in their attitudes towards the patient's symptoms and behaviour. Whereas high-EE relatives discount the patient's psychotic experiences as 'nonsense', 'it's just your imagination', or 'the doctor says you're mad', low-EE relatives acknowledge the reality of the patient's experiences. However, they make it clear that they do not share these experiences.

The coping strategies they have developed include:

(a) *time out* – for example, a mother whose son would get very tense with her at times would suggest that he take the dog out for a walk;

(b) *distraction* – for example, a mother whose daughter would get agitated by references to herself on television would ask her to go into the kitchen and make a cup of tea;

(c) *reality testing* – for example, a father whose son claimed that there were microphones in the door knobs gave him a screwdriver and asked him to dismantle the knob in order to check it;

(d) *protection of personal/psychological space* – for example, a wife whose husband argued with his voices in front of her told him she knew he could not help responding to the voices but could he please do it in another room.

Many of the strategies developed spontaneously by low-EE relatives have now been endorsed by the success of cognitive approaches to delusions and hallucinations (e.g. Fowler et al, 1995).

Targeting interventions

In our research and in our clinical work we have selected families in which at least one member is rated as 'high EE'. This does not imply that low-EE families are not in need of help, only that high-EE families have a higher priority, and we have to be selective when trained therapists are in short supply. With our colleagues we have established two national training centres, in Manchester and London (the Thorn Initiative). A key aim of the initiative is to develop satellite training centres to make this form of help available on a national basis to all families who could benefit. Currently six satellite centres are running and another six are in the process of being established. Although the training courses were originally limited to psychiatric nurses, they are now open to any psychiatric professional who has had sufficient experience of working with people suffering from psychosis.

Training in the use of the Camberwell Family Interview (CFI; Brown & Rutter, 1966) and the EE rating scales is not part of the course, since we view these techniques as mainly for use in research studies. However, trainees are instructed in the use of the Krawiecka–Goldberg scale for assessing symptoms (Krawiecka et al, 1977) and the Social Functioning Scale (Birchwood et al, 1990) so that they can monitor the progress of their clients.

Most mental health services have to concentrate resources on the families in greatest need. In the absence of ratings of relatives' EE, such families can be identified by the following rules of thumb:

(a) relatives living with patients who relapse more often than once a year despite being compliant with maintenance neuroleptics;
(b) relatives who frequently contact staff for reassurance or help;
(c) families in which there are repeated arguments that lead to verbal or physical violence, and any family that calls in the police;
(d) a single relative, usually the mother, looking after a person with schizophrenia on her own.

The treatment model

Our model of treatment is highly specific and consists of a psycho-educational component and a structured family approach, with an emphasis on cognitive–behavioural techniques. It is known that educating relatives about the illness and working with them to tackle some of their problems will attenuate their critical or overinvolved behaviour, and hence help to prevent relapses (see, for example, Leff et al, 1982, 1985, 1989, 1990; Tarrier et al, 1988).

The following are the basic assumptions and philosophy of the treatment model:

(a) Schizophrenia is conceptualised as a condition with a biological basis. A stress–vulnerability model is used to explain how, in a vulnerable person, stresses such as unexpected life changes might bring on the illness or a relapse.
(b) Instead of the relatives being blamed, they are enlisted as therapeutic agents, in order to help the patients. Furthermore, the burden and stress of living with a person with schizophrenia are taken seriously.
(c) There is an emphasis on openness and working in partnership with the family. Information about the illness is shared. In doing so the therapists also admit that there is a lot about the illness that is not known. Collaboration is elicited by mutual work on the setting of goals, priorities and tasks.
(d) Families are seen to have needs and strengths. A positive approach is used to build on a family's strengths in order to tackle their problems.

(e) The psychosocial family intervention described here is offered as part of a package, in conjunction with drugs and out-patient management. There is no attempt to substitute traditional management with family treatment.

Differences between our approach to work with families and that of others

People began to work with families in the early 1950s. At first, the focus was on families caring for a relative with schizophrenia, but it soon broadened to include families with a relative with any of the whole range of psychiatric conditions. The earliest work was based on psychoanalytic theory; however, in recent years this approach has been eclipsed by the rise of systemic family therapy.

The work we describe in this manual belongs to neither of these schools, although it has borrowed ideas and techniques from the systemic approach. The differences between our mode of working and that of others are worth spelling out.

The disease concept of schizophrenia

Some psychoanalytic theories trace the origin of schizophrenia to disturbed parent–child relationships. Within this tradition, schizophrenia is viewed as a purely psychological disturbance that is explicable in terms of the disturbance induced in the child by the parents.

The systemic view is rather different, since schizophrenia is seen as the presentation by one member of a 'mad' family situation. The madness characterises the whole family system, in which one member is 'chosen' to present it to the professional. This person is often referred to as 'the designated patient', with the implication that the pathology lies in the whole family.

In contrast to the above approaches, we consider that schizophrenia has a biological basis in brain dysfunction and can occur in families that are functioning perfectly well.

The role of the family

It is evident from the above that both psychoanalytic and systemic theories implicate the family in the causation of schizophrenia. We consider that families do not exert a causal influence, although they can modify the course of the illness.

The aim of therapy

In both psychoanalytic and systemic family therapy, the aim is to correct presumed family dysfunction. The family is consequently the client of the therapists. We do not view the family as in need of treatment. Hence we avoid calling our interventions 'family therapy'. Our aim is to help the family to cope better with a relative who is suffering from a specific illness. We see the family as an ally in treating the person with schizophrenia.

The role of insight

In psychoanalytic, but not systemic, family therapy, the insight of the therapist is fed back to the family in the form of interpretations to effect change. Although there is value in a psychodynamic understanding of family relationships, we do not offer interpretations to the family. We have found that they fail to produce change in families living with a person with schizophrenia.

The role of the therapists

In traditional psychoanalytic therapy, the therapist avoids answering direct questions and does not offer advice. We set out to give the family information, advice and guidance. However, we do not expect the family to be a passive recipient of these. Instead, we encourage the family to take an active part in discussing the information provided and to work with us to find solutions to their problems. In addition, we are active on behalf of the family in negotiating with various services. This would not be undertaken by a traditional psychoanalyst, although a systemic therapist might work with external agencies as part of the larger system within which the family operates.

General interpersonal effectiveness

The model of therapy used here emphasises the importance of rapport (a good and harmonious working relationship) with families. To be consistent with our family work model, the therapists should never criticise or blame the family. Apart from being an undesirable role model for the relatives, any criticism is likely to be passed on to the patient. The Rogerian principles of therapists being warm, empathic and genuine are seen as crucial for effective working with families. Therapists should show adequate warmth towards individuals in families – they are human beings in need of help. Empathy is defined as the ability to understand accurately the perspectives of other people. It is different from sympathy, which is the sharing of or having compassion for another individual's pain. It could be argued that too much sympathy could make therapists lose their objectiveness and hence ability to help. Furthermore, therapists should be genuine, open and sincere with families. Any unrealistic or unmet promise would be judged by families as insincere.

Therapists should not adopt an authoritarian attitude or impose the official view of schizophrenia on families. There is an important distinction between making factual statements about what we know regarding the illness and being insensitive and authoritarian. Moreover, it is important to elicit families' views regularly to gain their collaboration. Family members' feelings, experiences, strengths and needs should be respected. Being able to stay together, particularly when there are tensions and conflicts, should be viewed as a strength. Families' past or present attempts to cope, no matter how undesirable they may be to the therapists, should be respected as their best effort to cope, given their resources.

The premise of our model is that these interpersonal qualities are necessary but not sufficient for a good therapeutic outcome. The techniques described in this treatment model are enhanced when carried out in a good therapeutic relationship. If there is not such a relationship, therapy can be seen as robotic, and families would think that the therapists do not care about or understand them. Considerable skill is required to convey a good and caring professional attitude. The degree of warmth and genuineness being expressed by the therapists is important. But one could argue that the amount of warmth and genuineness perceived by individual family members is more important. The way to find out is by asking for regular feedback. Perhaps one of the best ways to learn how to convey these qualities initially is to observe how more experienced colleagues do it.

Support group for therapists

Work with families living with schizophrenia is emotionally demanding. We have found that therapists benefit from having a support group of their peers which meets about once a month. This may not always be feasible, but should be given high priority since it provides peer group supervision, as well as acting as a think tank to work on difficult problems.

Summary

We conceptualise schizophrenia as having a biological basis that makes the patient sensitive to stress. Consequently, our therapeutic approach involves drug treatment in conjunction with family work. Families are seen as partners of the therapists in an alliance to help the patients. We do not blame the relatives for the illness, nor do we view the family as in need of treatment. However, looking after someone with schizophrenia is demanding work, and the relative's emotional response to the patient can lead to worsening of the symptoms. Criticism, hostility and overinvolvement from the relatives are difficult for the patient to deal with. On the other hand, relatives who show warmth to the patient can improve the outcome of the illness. Therapists also should be warm and empathic but in addition need to work actively with the family on their problems. Therapists benefit from having their own support group.

Part II

Practical issues in family work

CHAPTER 2

Engaging the family

The intervention is a package composed of a variety of types of work with the family. The three basic components are:
(a) an education programme;
(b) family sessions in the home;
(c) a relatives' group.

The intervention begins with the education programme; then family sessions are arranged. Additionally, relatives may be invited to attend a group, which can be run in parallel with the family sessions.

It is very likely that a family will be reluctant to engage in treatment sessions. There may be a history of unhelpful previous professional contact, actual or perceived. Relatives may feel blamed for the illness and worry that treatment will pinpoint this. There is often a very real fear that any change will make things worse, not better, and that the status quo, even with all its problems, is, after all, to be preferred. Finally, and especially after many years of living with a person with schizophrenia, there may be an atmosphere of resignation, a feeling that 'nothing can be done', so that any help will be a waste of everyone's time.

Clinical example
This illustrates a family's dissatisfaction with previous professional contacts and a sense of resignation. (In all the clinical examples, T stands for therapist, M and F for mother and father, H and W for husband and wife, and P for the patient.)
M. They let him out because he was malicious. That's what they told me. I mean they don't have to deal with him if they choose to. But guess where he went? He came straight home and I had to deal with it all. I rang up the ward and that girl said she was scared of him. I mean there were so many of them and they were scared. What about me? And they gave him a week's supply of drugs. This is the first time they did that since my last showdown with them. If he takes an overdose this time, I would hold the hospital responsible. I sometimes wonder if things are ever going to get any better.

We do know that people are more likely to accept help at a time of crisis, for example after an admission to hospital. If there is an adamant refusal, therapists may have to wait until a future crisis to try again.

Engaging the family is the first task: unless a family's reluctance to engage is tackled, then however skilled the intervention, it will not be taken up.

Therapists must be aware that every professional contact with the family, each telephone call or chat in the corridor, is part of this engagement process and it should not be done in an offhand way.

It helps to remember that most families will have many needs, and that if they can be engaged, then these are likely to be addressed. On the therapists' part, engagement consists of offering positive, pleasant, polite contact, while sharing appropriate care and concern for the family's problems. This must be offered consistently, despite a family's negative response. They may refuse contact, avoid appointments, turn up late or not at all, or make it difficult to arrange a firm time; when a time has finally been arranged a crucial family member may miss the meeting.

There is an advantage in beginning with the education programme, since the therapists are offering something families are often desperate for – information. Furthermore, the fact that the therapists are prepared to make the effort to visit the home in order to give the family information aids the process of engagement.

The only situations in which we have found it impossible to engage a family have been when patients have been so suspicious of the therapist, or have specific paranoid ideas, that they refuse to allow access to the relative. One wife was terribly jealous of any contact her husband had, and the family felt too worried to accept a visit. These worries have to be respected and help offered later, when the ideas may be less firmly held.

Strategies

The general strategy for engagement is to offer positive experiences of contact, at the pace which the family will allow. Persistence is often necessary, as refusal at first contact is common. Being flexible as to the time and place of a visit, not becoming angry when arrangements break down, and continuing to offer another meeting will often enable enough trust to be built up for the family to risk a meeting.

It may be helpful to meet informally before family work begins, so that a family feels they have some prior knowledge of who the therapists are and what they are like. Sometimes, of the two therapists (see Chapter 4), one at least will have had contact before. One may have met a patient while he or she was acutely ill in hospital, so that the patient may be able to introduce therapist to the rest of the family. A relative, while visiting, may have been greeted by a therapist. It is important that these early, informal contacts are pleasant and reassuring. It is not going to help a family engage if there have been previous angry or hostile exchanges.

Families who refuse

If the family continues to refuse contact, there may come a point when this has to be accepted, and help offered at a later stage. However, there are some strategies therapists should try first.

If neither of the therapists knows the family, they should try to get introduced informally by a trusted third party, who can be reassuring about their involvement. It can help if they have some short statements in mind as to their reason for wanting to work with the family: "We would like to see how you're all getting on now that John is coming home soon", "We want to find out how things are at the moment and see if we can help you with any problems that may arise".

Sometimes it can help to meet the family singly; a first meeting may be with one relative alone. Once this contact has been made, it is important that the therapists make it clear that they would like to meet all those who have reasonably close contact with the patient (live in the same house, visit frequently, are key persons such as parents or partners). Separate letters to all relatives stating the time and date of the next meeting have been found to be useful. It cannot be assumed that family members will pass on messages, and an individually addressed letter is likely to be received and read. It is important for therapists to convey to the family that it would be helpful for everyone to attend who is or has been involved in the caring for the patient.

The most usual family member to show reluctance to participate in meetings is the father. Again, a separate letter to him, encouraging attendance and stating the time and date of the next meeting can be helpful. Occasionally the patient will not engage. Usually this is connected to acute phases of the illness, but sometimes a patient will feel that listening to relatives' complaints will not be productive. Make it clear to the patient that everyone will have a say in a family meeting and that all problems can be aired and listened to. It is then important to stick to these rules.

For some families, despite all efforts, only part of the family system will engage. It is important for therapists to work with whoever will attend; they can become advocates and persuade other family members to join in. It is worth keeping the channels open and continuing to ask if absent family members would like to join meetings. Often, after many months, they will. However, even if only one or two family members accept the help, it should still be offered; it is possible, though often more difficult, to effect change through part of the family system, and therapists should always be prepared to do so.

Maintaining families in treatment

Once the family has come to attend the first family session, one of the main tasks for the therapists is to maintain them in treatment. Some families might have had bad experiences with help from professionals in the past and be sceptical about the present offer of help. Others might hold unrealistic expectations of therapy. Families who have tried to cope for years might feel pessimistic about the future, but have decided to find out what the therapists have to offer. Hence it is extremely important to explore the family's past experience of professional help, their expectation of therapy this time, and their pessimism. It is a delicate balance between infusing hope and conveying what realistically can be expected from therapy. Empathy, warmth and genuineness help. In addition, the therapists should convey the message that this type of family work has repeatedly been found to prevent relapses, and spell out that any change is likely to be gradual. They should also express their willingness to work with the family.

Sometimes families will not acknowledge any positive changes. Therapists are cautioned not to argue and attempt to prove their therapeutic efficacy, as these families are likely to respond by showing the therapists that they are wrong. Instead, the therapists should reiterate that changes are slow. Attempts should be made to understand why these families are frightened to admit that change has occurred.

During treatment, therapists should make clear the purpose of behavioural goals and relate them from time to time to what the family want to achieve ultimately, so that they understand the small steps involved. Regular feedback, either verbally or in writing (e.g. 'Helpful Aspects of Therapy' forms – see Appendix 2), helps to elicit from families the way in which they see the treatment is going. Another important aspect of therapy is to hold regular reviews with families to explore how they feel about treatment. Any dissatisfaction or pessimism can then be dealt with before families decide to end treatment prematurely.

Summary

Families are likely to be difficult to engage in treatment. Be aware of this and be prepared to be persistent, and to continue to offer help even if it is initially rejected. We would always try to work with part of the family and aim to engage the others in due course. Initial contact may be informal or during a crisis, but always needs to be as pleasant and helpful as possible. Reminding families that progress will be slow helps to maintain them in treatment.

CHAPTER 3

Being a therapist, not a guest

Social pressures

The fact that sessions are often held in patients' homes rather than in a professional location needs special consideration. People who come to see professional staff in their own offices accept the unwritten rules that govern professional consultations. By contrast, staff visiting a home, particularly when they ask to see the whole family, are in an ambiguous position. Are they to be treated as professionals or guests? The family may wish to treat them as guests for a number of reasons. They are likely to be grateful that the staff have made the effort to come to them and often express their gratitude by offering hospitality. The influence of culture should not be ignored in this area. In some societies great importance is given to the idea of the guest as a person to be honoured and respected. It should be recognised that families from different cultural backgrounds will differ in their attitudes towards a member of staff entering their home.

Family members may try to turn the visit into a social occasion to avoid working on the problems they experience. Be wary of these attempts, as it is easy to be diverted from the main purpose of the visit. It is understandably more comfortable to settle into a social role than to steer the family firmly in the direction of hard work.

Family members are often socially isolated from friends and relatives outside the home. The therapists may be seen as welcome company to relieve loneliness. This can also lead to pressure from family members to adopt a social role.

The therapists' presence in the home will offer them an opportunity to change the family's style of interaction. Some relatives manage to transform the home into a mini-hospital, in which family life is entirely focused on the patient's illness. The therapists may be the first people from the outside world to enter this atmosphere for a long time. They can offer the family the prospect of a different lifestyle, which is less grim and more pleasurable.

Forms of address

The problems around establishing a therapeutic role start at the very beginning, when the therapists introduce themselves to the family. How should they refer to themselves – by their first name, their surname, or both, and should they use a professional title (e.g. doctor) if they have one? How should they address family members – Mr and Mrs so and so, or first names?

There are no hard-and-fast rules, and therapists should adopt a style with which they are comfortable. However, there are a few guidelines. The two co-therapists need to establish an egalitarian relationship with each other and will want to talk to each other and refer to each other by name in front of the family. They will certainly want to address each other directly by first name, and it will appear odd and unnatural if they refer to each other by surname or title when talking to the family. Furthermore, if one of the pair is a doctor, the use of titles will emphasise an inequality between them that could impede attempts to empower disadvantaged family members.

When working with a parental family, one of the aims will be to reinforce intergenerational boundaries and the authority of the parents. This can be helped by addressing the parents as Mr and Mrs so and so. They will certainly refer to their son or daughter by their first name, so the therapists will need to follow suit. Parents may ask the therapists to call them by their first names, in which case it would be churlish to refuse. With a married couple the therapists should begin by using Mr and Mrs but should switch to first names if requested.

Greeting and parting

At the beginning of a session, when the therapists enter the patient's home, it is customary to exchange pleasantries. However, this should not be allowed to go on too long. The therapists need to get down to the business of the visit within the first few minutes. A good way to start is to ask a general question about how things have been since the last visit. The therapists should then work their way round to asking about the task that was set at the end of the previous session (see Chapter 8).

Sessions should last a specified period (usually an hour), and the family should be informed of this. The duration of the sessions should be kept to reasonably closely, but not rigidly. The therapists need to work towards getting the family to agree on a homework task by the end of the session. On leaving there is likely to be another exchange of pleasantries, but the therapists must make sure that all family members are aware of the date and time of the next session.

Turning off the television

Often, on arrival in a family's living room, the television will be on. It is essential that it is turned off if a family meeting is to proceed. Some families use the television as company, or even as 'wallpaper', and claim that it will not interfere with a meeting. However, even if the sound is turned down, visual images are extremely distracting and will capture the attention of everyone present. Before sitting down, if a polite request is made to turn off the television, all families we have ever worked with have done so.

Tea and biscuits

Some families regularly offer tea or coffee during a session, while with others this may happen from time to time. The therapists should start by assuming that the offer of a hot drink is customary and innocuous. There is usually no harm in accepting, and it may help the family feel that they are doing something to express their gratitude. However, the timing of the offer should be carefully considered. It may occur at a point in the session when it is clearly diversionary. In this case the therapists should thank the family member but ask if it could be postponed.

Another useful strategy can be used in a parental family in which the mother always makes the drinks. The patient can be asked to take on the task from time to time, thus preventing the mother's avoidance tactics and giving the patient an opportunity to demonstrate his/her competence.

Biscuits are often offered along with tea or coffee, which is acceptable, but some family members have been known to bake cakes especially for the therapists' visits. This has to be judged within the cultural context of the family, and if considered to be excessive should be politely but firmly discouraged.

Clinical example
We made regular visits to a Greek Cypriot mother and her ill daughter. Each time we came the mother had baked a large cake for us, from which she cut us each a very large slice. When we protested that the slices were too much for us, she cut them smaller, but at the end of the visit wrapped up the rest of the cake and presented it to us. We decided that there was no way of avoiding this traditional hospitality without upsetting our clients.

Alcoholic drinks should never be accepted.

Personal questions

Personal questions to the therapists may represent genuine curiosity or may be another way of socialising the visit. While refusal to answer any personal questions is likely to give an impression of rudeness, therapists should be wary of going into any detail about their personal lives. Failure to observe caution will open the way to increasing socialisation of the therapists' visits and may undermine working relationships.

Taking control

There are some circumstances in which the therapists need to exert a degree of control over the session. These include situations of open conflict, which are painful for the family members involved and are counter to the aims of the therapy. Another example is when the therapists wish to change the seating arrangements. In both these examples the therapists are required to take control over what is happening. Beginners often feel reluctant to take such a directive role in the family's own home. However, it is necessary to develop sufficient confidence in the value of these interventions to take control of the family from time to time, with the appreciation that eventually the family will learn to control situations themselves.

Summary

Working in a patient's home subjects therapists to unaccustomed social pressures. Therapists must ensure that they are able to maintain a working relationship with the family, while avoiding being uncivil. The television must always be turned off.

CHAPTER 4

Co-therapy

For this form of family work we do recommend that therapists work in pairs. We have always found it helpful to have two people, to plan the family session, discuss what happened and decide what to do next. During a session it is an advantage to have one therapist observing while the other is talking, and vice versa. However, working with a co-therapist means that there is a professional relationship; this has to be constructive and any problem looked at to prevent difficulties.

Modelling

A pair of therapists provides a model for the family. Two people are trying to work together to improve things – they may not agree and they may not work in the same way. The way these differences are acknowledged and resolved may be the first indication that the family has had for many years that different viewpoints can be discussed. Modelling negotiating skills is a useful aspect of co-therapy. Acknowledging and discussing differences openly can help the family to learn how to do this without anger. Therapists should not try to do it, however, unless they know that they will manage it positively. Many families have been caught in repetitive and conflict-generating patterns that they cannot sort out. Therapists must make sure that they do not do the same.

Trust

Working with someone else means that the relationship has to incorporate trust and cooperation: therapists have to feel comfortable enough with their co-therapists to trust their judgement and be able to reinforce what they do or suggest. This is the model to aim for. There is no point in a therapist starting work with a family with a partner whom she/he intensely dislikes or disapproves of. Therapists must respect each other's skills and be able to offer support to each other. However, even with a trusted partner there will be times, during family sessions, when a therapist will feel angry, dislike what was done or feel his/her skills were neglected. They should use a debriefing session to air these feelings and sort them out. If necessary, outside supervision or help should be sought. Therapists should not let actively negative feelings between them surface during the session. It is likely that they themselves would be recreating family conflicts, and that the anger and dislike are reflections of the family dysfunction. The therapists' role is to defuse conflict and not to perpetuate it.

Forming alliances

Working collaboratively and constructively does not imply that the therapists both have to do the same thing in a session. Often it is helpful for them to work together, to take up and agree points the other has made. There are other times when it can be helpful for them to work with separate parts of the family system. They may want to enforce generation boundaries, so one of them will work with the parents, voicing their concerns, making sure their view is heard, while the other may work with the patient, acknowledging the problems, helping him/her put ideas across. These 'alliances' can ensure that parts of the family are not alienated or neglected. However, such alliances should be flexible. It should be possible to change them if necessary. Otherwise family members can feel that only one therapist understands them.

Working on separate tasks

Sometimes it can be helpful to split tasks. When giving the education one therapist has to read it and the other can usefully pick up the problems and emotional issues that the family raises. One therapist may have particular expertise that the family asks for – information on benefits, on medication, on decisions that the 'team' has been involved in; it is helpful to use this knowledge and for one therapist to supply the answer.

Planning sessions

Before a session starts, the therapists should take some time together to plan the detail of what they will do. The important thing here is to have a small number of joint aims and some idea of how to achieve them. Sessions can never be planned absolutely; families may have a pressing problem to discuss, which will take priority. It is also necessary for therapists to be spontaneous and react to the nuances of family functioning, so that families know that they are listening and responding to their problem and not to some predetermined list. However, it is helpful for therapists to decide who will start the session, what they will try to achieve and when it will finish.

Support during the session

During a session, it is likely that the therapists will feel stuck at some stage. They may not know what to do. They may suddenly feel that the discussion is missing the point or that a difficult emotional issue has been raised. It is useful for the co-therapists to use each other at this point in the session. It is helpful if they admit openly that they have a problem, to think aloud and to consult with each other over what should happen next. This consultation is a more overt part of what should be happening between them; they should both be aware of each other's input and be able to check whether a particular suggestion is the one to pursue.

Sometimes it may be necessary for therapists to 'rescue' each other. One therapist may be diverted by the family, put off the point or led into an irrelevant discussion. The other therapist must be alert to these possibilities and be prepared to make an intervention that pulls the family back to the task or aim of the session.

Debriefing

At the end of a session therapists should make sure they leave time to discuss what happened. If one or both rushes off, it can sometimes leave quite intense feelings of concern or anxiety. They should make sure that these concerns are brought out immediately and dealt with in some way, and that a decision is made about the next meeting.

Summary

Working with a co-therapist is recommended, but requires that the relationship is positive and constructive, and models negotiating skills. Two people working together allows alliances to be made and tasks to be split. The relationship requires trust for any conflict to be dealt with, if necessary using outside supervision. Co-therapy is more effective if sessions are planned together beforehand, therapists support each other during a session, and sufficient time is allowed for debriefing afterwards.

CHAPTER 5

Offering education

Clinical example
This illustrates relatives' need for information. This woman's daughter had been ill for eight years and was on biweekly injections.
M.   You see, when I went to the doctor for the doctor to tell me what it is, I expected the doctor to say "Oh, Coral suffers from schizophrenia. You must watch her behaviour pattern; you must be careful because she suffers from this. She will do this or she will do that – whatever." But nothing. Nobody said anything to me. Nobody.

The education programme

The material is in the form of a booklet published by the National Schizophrenia Fellowship (reproduced in amended form as Appendix 1 to this volume). The topics are: symptoms of schizophrenia, its cause and course, and its treatment.

The education is given in two sessions in the home and two sections of the booklet are worked through on each occasion. It is usual to give the programme while the patient is still in hospital, so that only the relatives are present. A booklet is left with the relatives to go over in their own time. Patients should be actively involved in an education programme, either on their own or with the relatives. If the patient is to be educated with the relatives, some preparation may be needed, particularly a discussion of the diagnosis and why it is being made.

The material from the booklets is read out exactly as it is written; however, it is interspersed with comments which tailor it to the patient's particular situation. In order to be able to do this, the therapist has to become familiar with the patient's range of symptoms and the family history beforehand. For example, "'He may hear voices talking to him or about him.' I think that has happened to John, hasn't it?" " 'Many arguments can arise over his personal cleanliness.' I think, though, that John has always kept himself neat and clean."

The therapist should tell the family members before starting that there will be plenty of time to ask questions and should pause after each statement to allow the family to respond. Some families will need encouragement to ask questions, make statements or voice their disagreement with various items of information. The therapist must be prepared to enter into discussion with the family and to clarify the information in the booklets, but will also need to listen to and try to understand the family's view. On no account should the therapist attempt to impose the 'official' view on the family. Some families never accept the diagnosis of schizophrenia, in which case the therapists need to agree with the family to differ over diagnosis. This need not prevent them from working with the family.

Clinical example
This illustrates the importance of listening to the family's view and not imposing the 'official' view.

T. That's what we call it, schizophrenia. What do you call your problem, David?

P. Em, I don't know. I don't know what it is. Depression I suppose that's what it's called. If the professor is saying to me... I mean, he didn't say to me that you've got schizophrenia. He just said you are ill, or he just said he thought you had an illness. But, em, if he had said to me that you had schizophrenia, I would be quite concerned because, you know, I need to be treated for it. It seems to be more of a dangerous illness than what I seem to have at the moment. I really needed to be in hospital longer or be under his guidance a little bit longer. But he hadn't said that.

T. Your illness is similar to what we would term schizophrenia. Now you may have a different term for that or a different name. That's fine. But I think it may be useful to go through some of the information we have about schizophrenia. I think there are often a lot of fantasies or things that people have heard about schizophrenia that actually aren't true in many ways. So should we press on?

P. But it doesn't seem that they are quite clear. It just seems that schizophrenia doesn't seem to have any kind of patterns. It's an illness that just affects people differently. And it may not be the same illness that causes schizophrenia. It just seems to be all over the place really. You might not get it again.

T. I suppose, like with most problems, you may get a core of things that you can say are principally the same or similar. But of course we are all individuals and the way that we respond to a particular illness is bound to be dependent on our individual personalities. And so the way that we become ill will be very different for everybody.

P. So it's down to the individual really, the illness.

The long-term process of education

The education programme is only the very beginning of a process of education which will continue throughout the meetings with the family. The family's view of the patient's condition is unlikely to change in response to the education sessions, but usually shifts gradually, over a year or so. Family members will repeatedly ask the same questions over a long time. The therapists need to be patient in repeating the same information and in negotiating with family members over the differences between their views of the patient's condition and the 'official' version. When a resolution of differences is achieved, the questions about that area usually cease. However, a new crisis will often precipitate a resurgence of questions. It must be recognised that even if family members accept most of the information, they rarely change their beliefs about causation.

The main topics

In each area of the education programme there are two main points that the therapist needs to emphasise. They are as follows:

(a) Causation
   (i) The family is not to blame for the illness.
   (ii) Inheritance plays a part, but there are other causes which have yet to be discovered.

(b) Negative symptoms
   (i) The negative symptoms are caused by the illness and are not under the patient's control.
   (ii) They do not generally respond to drugs but will gradually improve over one to two years.

(c) Positive symptoms
   (i) There is a great deal of individual variation in the positive symptoms.
   (ii) The experiences of delusions and hallucinations are real to the patient, and the relative should not dismiss them as 'imagination' or 'nonsense'.

(d) Prognosis
   (i) One in four people who develop schizophrenia will recover completely and remain well for years.
   (ii) Most of the remainder will improve and can lead relatively normal lives outside hospital.
   It is important to give the family hope.

(e) Treatment and management
   (i) The illness makes patients sensitive to stress, which should be reduced where possible in order to benefit both patient and relatives.
   (ii) Drugs help in the long term, but it is also important that the atmosphere is calm and predictable.

It is no use telling family members not to be critical or overinvolved. People cannot simply stop behaving in a particular way in response to advice, especially if they are driven by emotion. They will perceive this as criticism of themselves and it will make them less likely to engage with the intervention. The therapists will be working with them to help change these attitudes over a long period. However, it is important for the family to understand what the goals are, namely a calm rather than argumentative atmosphere, predictable rather than inconsistent attitudes, and support and tolerance rather than rejection.

After the second education session, the therapists offer to come regularly to help the family tackle the problems of everyday life with a person with schizophrenia.

Summary

Education about schizophrenia is given in two sessions in the relatives' home. It covers the causes, symptoms and prognosis of schizophrenia, and the treatment and management. It is tailored to the individual patient's symptoms and circumstances. It is only the beginning of a process of learning about the illness that continues throughout work with the family.

CHAPTER 6

Family sessions

Any social group has a structure. In families the structure is usually organised around parent–child and husband–wife relationships. These vary with era and culture; for instance, the conventional image of the father as the head of the household is disappearing among middle-class white people, whereas it remains intact in many Asian families in Britain. Furthermore, there is an increasing number of single-parent households in which the mother carries full parental responsibility. These variations have to be borne in mind when assessing the structure of the family therapists are going to work with (the cultural issues are discussed further in Chapter 22). There are some general guidelines that apply.

(a) When there are two parents, it is better if they can cooperate in the care of the children rather than having opposing views and practices.

(b) All members of a family should respect one another. The parents should respect the children's need to move towards independence. The children should respect the parents' need to live part of their lives separately from the children.

(c) Each family needs to decide what behaviour they find unacceptable and should be able to set limits to it.

Aims

The aims of family work will obviously differ for parental and marital families. When the patient lives with two parents, the aims are:

(a) To encourage cooperation between the mother and father so that they enhance each other's efforts rather than hindering them. The problems presented by schizophrenia are often very difficult and cannot be tackled effectively unless the parents work together. Furthermore, the person with schizophrenia is likely to exploit any divisions between the parents, as may any offspring.

(b) To maintain a balance of power between the parents so that they share responsibility for the patient equally.

(c) To strengthen the boundaries between parents and children so that the person with schizophrenia in particular can move towards independence.

(d) To release the parents from full-time caring so that they can spend some time away from the patient, and enjoy each other's company.

These aims have to be modified for single-parent households, in which it is usually the mother who is the carer. In this case a major aim is to develop or enhance links the mother has with people outside the household, in order to provide the emotional support she needs and to create an alternative focus of interest for the patient.

In marital households the aims are:

(a) To maintain a balance of power between the partners (this may be difficult if the patient is very disabled by schizophrenia, but it must be recognised that the illness can be a source of power in itself – relatives may be frightened of violence, whether realistically or not, and on a more mundane level the patient can exploit the sick role to evade responsibility).

(b) To enhance the couple's enjoyment of the relationship. This is usually possible, unless it was a loveless marriage in the first place.

(c) To help adjust the roles in the family so that the patient can find an area of competence and contribute to the well-being of the family. This might involve, for example, the wife going out to work while the husband looks after the children.

(d) To ensure that the partner gets some time off from caring.

Achieving the aims

This will be dealt with in detail throughout this manual, but it may be helpful to summarise the approaches here. They include the formation of alliances between the therapists and family members, modelling of cooperation and a balanced partnership by the co-therapists, setting tasks that bring the parents together and separate them from the children, exploring parental anxieties about separation from the children, giving each member an equal opportunity to speak, and helping patients to improve their competence and confidence.

Briefing and debriefing

Agreeing on the aims before a session and debriefing after it are important advantages of working with a co-therapist (see Chapter 4).

Summary

Work with families has to take into account the norms for family structure and roles that exist in particular social and cultural groups. However, there are general principles for therapists to follow, such as the need for family members to respect each other and to cooperate in attempting to improve the quality of their lives.

CHAPTER 7

Improving communication

The problems

Some families with a member who has schizophrenia communicate well, but others show disturbed patterns of communication which hinder useful work with them. Often this is the result of high levels of emotional tension and trying to cope with numerous problems, both of which produce a stream of talk that is difficult to interrupt. We have found that high-EE relatives talk more than low-EE relatives, although patients in the two types of family speak about the same amount. Many people with schizophrenia are unable to assert themselves, and so get left out of conversations. The members of such families have often lost the ability to listen to one another; their monologues become repetitive and are not modified by other people's responses.

A small minority of blood relatives express themselves in unusual ways which may impede communication. This characteristic is akin to the thought disorder sometimes found in schizophrenia and shows itself by illogical jumps in the flow of speech or a peculiar use of words. In a multicultural society some family members may not speak English as their first language, and allowance needs to be made for lack of fluency. If the language problem is pronounced, a translator should be used, or better still a therapist who is fluent in the relevant language.

Establishing the ground rules

A good way of improving communication is to lay down a set of ground rules early on in the family meetings, and to help the family members to respect them. They are as follows.

Only one person may speak at a time

This may appear obvious, but family members often speak over each other, sometimes carrying on parallel conversations with the two co-therapists.

Therapists can introduce this rule by saying that it is impossible for them to listen to two people at once and, as they are keen to hear what everyone has to say, it is necessary for only one person to talk at a time. It can take many sessions for the family to settle down to a regular observance of this rule, and the therapists will probably have to remind them of it repeatedly. This should be done firmly, but without criticising family members, for example "I'm sorry, we can only listen to one person at a time. Who is going to be first?"

Successful establishment of this rule means that family members have increased their self-control, both over speech and over the emotional pressure behind the speech. It also helps them to show more respect to each other.

Talk to the person, not about them

It is quite common for family members to talk about another person in the session, referring to them as 'he' or 'she', as though that person were not present. It is often patients who are referred to in the third person, particularly if they speak very little. It is surprisingly easy for therapists to slip into this practice unawares. It needs to be checked in family members whenever it occurs, because it makes the person referred to feel as though she or he was not really present. This is particularly problematic for people with schizophrenia, who often have a fragile sense of self. Moreover, it may be particularly uncomfortable for patients who are experiencing third-person auditory hallucinations.

Say something along the lines of: "We would like to establish a rule that if anyone wants to say something about a person in the room, they should speak directly to them." Family members will need frequent reminding of this rule. It can be helpful to say, "What you have just said is very important. Would you like to tell your husband directly?"

Another advantage of direct communication is that it tones down the expression of negative emotions. It is much more difficult to say directly to someone "You're a very lazy person" than it is to say "He's a very lazy person".

Speaking time should be shared out equally

It is quite common for one relative to take the lion's share of the conversation, to the exclusion of others, particularly the patient. The therapists need to explain that it is important to hear the views of each family member. They have to keep the more loquacious members in check and encourage the reticent ones. However, stopping relatives in the middle of a sentence could be seen as rudeness. Therapists have to develop a style which is firm but tactful, for example "I know you have something important to say Mr Brown, but we would like to give your wife a chance to say something too, and we will come back to you later." The use of humour can sometimes sugar the pill.

Occasionally families cannot be kept in check this way and a more formal structure is required, for example giving each family member two minutes to talk.

The patient is usually the most disadvantaged in conversations and tends to get left out. This can be dealt with by giving the patient time in which to speak during which no other family member may interrupt. The patient may experience this as an uncomfortable pressure to contribute. In this case the therapists can reassure the patient that there is no need to speak at all during this time, but that everyone else will keep quiet and listen just in case the patient wants to say something.

Listening skills

In addition to the ground rules, it is important for the therapists to improve family members' listening skills. This is partly achieved by preventing talking over and interrupting, but it can also be encouraged more actively. It can be helpful to point out to one family member that another is saying something important, and to ask him/her to listen carefully. When the speaker has finished talking, the listener can be asked to repeat what was said in his/her own words. This is a good check on how well or badly family members are communicating with each other.

Each person's point of view, however poorly expressed, should be valued by the therapists. This helps everyone to feel that they are contributing to the session. If someone is speaking in a muddled way, the therapists can say that they are not quite clear about the message and ask for clarification. If necessary, the therapists can help a person towards a clearer expression of what he/she wishes to convey.

Summary

Communication can be improved by establishing ground rules. Only one person should speak at a time. Family members should speak directly to each other. Everyone should get a fair share of speaking time. In addition, family members often need encouragement to listen actively to each other.

CHAPTER 8

Task setting

Setting a realistic list of goals

One of the most important tasks therapists have to undertake is to help families to deal with the many problems they may have. These problems may be a result of having to live with a member of the family suffering from a major mental illness or due to other factors in the family. Often intervention is in the form of problem solving. An essential ingredient of successful problem solving in therapy is to have an unambiguous list of goals. Problems defined vaguely or globally lead to vague or impossible solutions. Just as sometimes therapists ask a relative who is being hostile to reframe and specify a global criticism – such as changing "He is so untidy" to "I would like him to clear up part of his bedroom" – so they have to ask the family to spell out goals in concrete terms that they and the family can work on. This may sound easier than it is in reality. However, it is an essential step in therapy. The list of specific goals can be drawn up over several sessions, but it will anyway be constantly updated as therapy progresses.

Setting an agenda and prioritising

One of the characteristics of working with families with a member who has schizophrenia is the unpredictability the illness can bring. Hence therapy should be flexible, to accommodate any new or urgent problems. However, therapists should not be diverted into 'just putting out bushfires' session after session. A behavioural approach is particularly suited to this type of family work because it provides structure and continuity. The process is very much collaborative.

At the beginning of each session, therapists should elicit any new problems the family may have had since the last session. These should be considered in conjunction with continuing problems that remain unresolved. Each family member should be given a chance to voice problems and concerns. These in turn can be put on the agenda for negotiation and prioritising. It is often essential to focus on just one problem at a time. It is common for family members to divert therapists from their focus on a single problem by raising equally pressing problems. This must be resisted politely but firmly, with the explanation that progress can be made only by dealing with one problem at a time. Sometimes, as work on a particular problem is reaching a conclusion, irrelevant or diversionary topics are brought up, for example an offer to make tea. As before, the therapists need to insist on maintaining the focus.

Clinical example
This illustrates how to set an agenda and focus on one problem at a time.
M. It's not only a drink problem. It's the money side of it, borrowing, borrowing, borrowing. Like today he has nothing left from social security to give me. And it is a terrible habit you have got into. If I suddenly disappeared, you wouldn't know what to do.
T1. I think part of the problem here is that there are a lot of problems. There is the drinking, budgeting, laundry and the weekend. So what does cause the most tension do you think, Peter [the patient]?
M. Well maybe not to Peter but it does to me dear. It has got to a point that I just go along with him. What else can I do?
T2. Well the purpose of coming here is to perhaps look at the problems and put them in some sort of priority, some sort of order. Perhaps we should start with one. In dealing with one problem, we might make some impact on the others. Can we look at one and deal with one problem at a time?

The process of dealing with one thing at a time is not only realistic but also a good opportunity to 'role model' to the family how to solve problems. It would be advisable not to pick the most entrenched or difficult problem to deal with, at least initially, so that families can have some experience of success in therapy. All too often their experience will have been dominated by failure. It requires a lot of skill to persuade families to accept a less entrenched problem as the focus of therapy, as they will be inclined to think that their concerns and worries are being ignored. Not all problems have obvious solutions, at least initially. Once a small problem has been successfully tackled, the way to approach a bigger problem may become evident.

Negotiating solutions and agreeing on homework

Problems should be spelled out precisely and in enough detail to enable a solution to be found. Global descriptions such as "He is so lazy" should be reframed as "He does not get up till noon". Once a problem has been identified, each family member's views should be explored. Patients' experiences in relation to the problems are particularly valuable. A common problem is that the patient does not get up until the afternoon. There are three common causes: overmedication producing excessive sleepiness; reversal of the day–night rhythm – the patient stays up all night and sleeps during the day, sometimes as a means of avoiding social contact; there is nothing for the patient to get up for. Asking patients their times of going to sleep and waking up, and enquiring how they feel when they wake up, will pinpoint the cause. This example emphasises to the family the value of exploring the patient's experience of the problem.

Clinical example

This illustrates how the therapists should listen to everyone's view on the problem in order to understand it better.

T. Well it sounds to me like you are saying you don't want Peter to drink at the weekends and I am wondering, Peter, why you choose Saturday as your day to drink. Why don't you do it on a Thursday or a Monday, when you are not at your mother's house? You know she doesn't want you to drink?

P. Well I don't drink much on a Saturday. It's only four cans or something like that. It's usually because I have taken Sudafed in the day and it makes me hyper-tense in the evening. So if I take a drink it calms me down again. I think what I have got to do is stop taking the Sudafed and that will stop me drinking.

T. How about drinking at your mother's house? Could you do one or the other? Either you drink on Saturday and not go to your mother's house, or you go to your mother and not drink.

M. The fact is that Peter will change after a drink. And I've seen that change many, many a time. But I am not having it any more. I'm not, no way. I have gone beyond that.

T. Do you find that a reasonable request?

P. Yes, it's very reasonable.

T. Will you find that difficult?

P. Not because I change all that much. It's just that I find it difficult to talk to my mother when I have had a drink.

M. Maybe not, Peter, but you frighten me.

P. She can't have a conversation with me when I have had a drink because I am less inhibited. And she finds it difficult to get close to me when my inhibitions have gone. And plus the fact that there is a lot going on in my mind which could be potentially disturbing to her.

The therapists' next task is to encourage the family to express possible solutions to the problem, to look at the pros and cons of each solution, and to get the family to compromise and agree on a solution. Sometimes high-EE relatives find it impossible to think of a low-EE solution. It then falls to the therapist to suggest one. This is to be avoided if possible, as the family can always disqualify the therapist's suggestion by saying "You don't belong to the club. You don't have to look after a person with schizophrenia 24 hours a day, seven days a week." One of the advantages of a relatives' group is that low-EE solutions are likely to be thrown up by an assembly of relatives from different families (see Chapters 24 and 25).

Just as problems should be clearly defined, solutions should be operationalised in such a way that family members are clear about what each other's role is in carrying out the solution. Sometimes a relative's part is to do nothing, so that the patient can be given a chance to become more independent.

In negotiating the solution, therapists should also anticipate anything that might prevent it being effective. It could be that an overinvolved relative's anxiety is making the task too difficult, or simply that the solution is too ambitious. It may be helpful to refer to the task as 'an experiment'. Failure can then be construed as a badly designed experiment for which the family is not to be blamed.

Homework is important in therapy because it helps the family to generalise to the outside world what has been talked about in the session. The exact what, how, by whom, where and when of the task should be spelled out clearly, and in behavioural terms if possible. Sometimes it may be necessary for family members to write them down. Obtain agreement from all family members present to cooperate in trying the agreed solution. This acts as an insurance against sabotage by one or other member. To summarise, the steps are:

(a) specify in detail what the problem is;
(b) get everyone's view on the problem, particularly the patient's;
(c) elicit possible solutions;
(d) look at the pros and cons of each possible solution;
(e) compromise and agree on a desirable solution;
(f) anticipate any obstacles;
(g) spell out the exact what is to be done, how, by whom, where and when;
(h) assign the solution as an experiment as part of homework.

Clinical example

This is an example of how the therapists skilfully got the patient to agree on a solution that was workable and not too difficult for him.

T1. I was just wondering what can be done about your drinking or what you would like to do for the next weekend or for any weekend.

P. I want to stop it.

T1. I'm just wondering how practical it is.

P. I think it is pretty practical; I think I can manage it as long as I don't take the Sudafed.

T1. So if you don't take the Sudafed, you wouldn't take the alcohol?

P. Yes.

T2. My own feeling about that is that it's been a long-standing problem and it's not going to change overnight.

P. Yes.

T1. I am just wondering if we could try to work out something which is practical and possibly achievable, in terms of the first step, before we meet again.

P. Well can I make a promise to you that I'll not drink this week. I would feel very bad if I don't keep that promise. You're not forcing me into it – I'm volunteering it.

T1. No. But we want you to succeed at what we agree. There is no point in saying "I will never drink", because that is very, very hard for someone with your problem. We need to go very slowly.

T2. It's very good of you to offer the promise. It sounds very laudable and very constructive. But it is a matter of pitching it at the point which is practical for you to achieve rather than promising so much and perhaps not achieving it. Perhaps it's best to promise less but make it achievable. I think our task is to break things down to the point where you can do something which is achievable.

P. But I think I realise now that it's not on if I drink on a Saturday – from my own point of view more than my mother's point of view. I have a lot of feedback from elsewhere. I mean, I talk to a psychologist and he said you are poisoning yourself every time you take a drink. I think that has sunk in pretty deeply and that is something that is playing on my mind. So I think it's feasible for me to say I won't have a drink on a Saturday; I think that is a reasonable goal at the moment.

Then the therapists anticipated problems which could prevent the patient from being successful in his task.

Tl. So how could your mother help with this? Do you want to ask your mother if she could help anywhere?

P.   Well, I don't think she could. She could sit down and have a conversation with me. If I decided I wanted a drink, I could talk it through with her. But I don't think that would be a reasonable idea because then there is always the opportunity that I might be open for a drink if I could persuade her.

T2. And what about Saturday, how would you manage on Saturday? What's your routine normally?

P.   Well if I promised it here and now, I don't think I am going to break my word.

T2. But I think when people have a problem with drink, you need to sort of say "Well, I'm going to do this and this to keep myself occupied".

M.   He hasn't done it every Saturday night.

P.   I do some painting.

T2. But I think, Peter, you need to have in your head what you are going to do to compensate. Have you any ideas? I mean, you can't paint all day.

P.   Not all day, but I can't paint in the evening. If I have a drink I can't paint at all so it's a waste of time.

The following shows how the therapists engaged the mother to help.

T1. Have you any ideas [to mother]?

M.   Look at it this way, Peter. When you haven't spent all this money on beer, there is nothing to stop us going to the theatre. That's where we used to go.

T2. That would be nice.

M.   As long as you pay your share. I can't afford it for the two. But you're spending it on something constructive and not going to have the beer. If I've got to drink all those beers, it would be enough to make my head ache.

T2. I think it is important to praise Peter. He is doing well and likes going to the theatre, which you might enjoy together.

P.   Yeah.

T1. So do you want to plan that in now as part of this package, that Peter would not drink on Saturday and do some painting? What is planned in as well is the theatre trip on Saturday.

Checking up on homework

It is extremely frustrating for families to be given homework and for therapists not even to bother to find out how it has gone in the next session. Finding out about homework from the last session should always be on the agenda if homework has been agreed on. Enough time should be allocated to go through homework thoroughly. If the agreed solution has been successful, the therapists should positively reinforce the family members involved. Other family members should be encouraged to praise and value any change, no matter how small it is. This is important, as it provides a model for recognising that small changes are the aim and must not be devalued. Family members then should be encouraged to try the solution again and to practise it whenever the opportunity arises. They should also be encouraged to generalise the principle or the solution to other problems.

Clinical example

This illustrates how therapists may encourage relatives to praise and value any small changes.

T1. Just wondering how things have been since two weeks ago. The agreement was for John to look after his own washing. We were talking about you doing less for John as a way of possibly satisfying both views on your responsibilities. We agreed that John would do more, to reduce what you were doing for him.

M.   I don't think it's materialised yet, not at the moment. I think John's trying to bring less washing to me but he didn't do any last week, because of the worry I suppose. It's a bit peculiar what I'm going to say. But whatever he does in the day centre, the sheets and shirts are very screwed up. It's an awful job to iron them and get them back to normal again. I have a machine which I can do myself and they come out reasonably for ironing. Here they come out sort of really screwed up and it's hard work to iron them. So I don't know which is the better of two evils.

T2.   How do you feel John?

P.   Well I didn't really feel like coming in on the Wednesday. I have very little washing because I got most of it done the previous week. I took a few things around to my mother's on Friday. But tomorrow I shall be able to do it again.

T2.   You started to make an effort.

M.   Yes he makes an effort to do towels and things like that. But learn to put them straight John and you don't get all that bundled up. If you know what I mean.

T1.   So the first step appears to be that John attempts to do the washing. That's the first step.

M.   Yes, he's trying.

T2.   And then you know that you're trying to improve.

T1.   How are the results to you John, were they acceptable to you?

P.   Not really because I was shirking.

T1.   Shirking?

P.   Yes. I wasn't really putting a great effort into it last week. I felt down last week, so that had something to do with it. But I should imagine this week that I will be able to do it. Perhaps tomorrow. I think tomorrow.

M.   Well it's good to be occupied. That's good – it helps me a bit.

Sometimes, despite the ingenuity and preparations of the therapists and the family, the solution may not work. This is part of therapy, and therapists should not feel angry or become despondent. Therapists should find out exactly what happened and why nothing was attempted if that was the case. Sometimes an unsuccessful intervention can be just as useful in the long run, since it can elucidate much about the family and its members. On no account should therapists blame the family or become angry with them. Therapists should accept responsibility for any failure. "The task was set too soon or was too difficult", "The experiment was poorly designed" and "The family is not ready for it yet" are some good ways to avoid blaming the family. Therapists should 'role model' how to deal with failures, which are part of life. The problem should be looked at again or a new problem chosen. Individual family members' views should be listened to and a new solution should be agreed upon, taking into account the obstacles causing the failure. This starts the whole process over again.

Summary

Agreeing on a list of goals, setting an agenda, prioritising, agreeing on solutions and assigning homework are all very much part of a collaborative process. Each family member's views and feelings should be elicited in turn. They should be listened to carefully and respected. The process of therapy is just as important as the content. It is particularly therapeutic to make sure the patient's views are listened to, no matter how passive or withdrawn the patient might be. This may be the only opportunity for the family to listen to each other's views with a constructive aim. Overinvolved relatives, who may have a tendency to think they know the patient's views or feelings without asking the patient, should be shown that it is important to ask and listen to the patient. This can help foster respect for patients as individuals, with their own thoughts and feelings. A lot of skill is required, as well as a clear idea of goals and techniques.

CHAPTER 9

Dealing with emotional upset: general issues

The variety of emotional responses

We know that living with schizophrenia gives rise to a wide variety of emotional responses. Families may deny there is a problem, particularly at the beginning of an illness. They may try hard to say that all difficulties are in the past and that problems will not recur. They will nonetheless probably have many negative emotions: relatives are likely to feel angry; they may sometimes be rejecting and wish the patient were not living with them, or that the patient would leave.

Relatives who are parents are almost certain to feel guilty and in some way to blame for the problems. They will often respond by sacrificing their own time and energy, offering care and protection, and trying to make things better. Some relatives may take this to extremes and attempt to do everything, to take over all the roles and treat the patient as a child again, not as an autonomous adult. In the short term, while the illness is florid, this can be a helpful reaction. In the long term, it impedes recovery because a patient has nothing to gain by an inappropriate, or childish, sick role in the family, and is likely both to lose skills and to become overdemanding.

Another emotion commonly experienced is a feeling of loss. There are two kinds of loss that may have to be faced. One is almost like a bereavement, and is the loss of the person who existed before the illness (see epigraph on p. v): the familiar relative seems to have been replaced by a stranger. The other is a loss of expectation, ambitions, hopes of achievement, potential career and autonomy. Both types of loss may involve an inability to accept how the patient is now. Patients themselves may well have had to cope with loss of their old self, of skills, of a job, of relationships, of a role in the community. These losses are often accompanied by reduced confidence and a worry about trying new things. Both relatives and patient may be frightened of change in case problems return, and they may not be sure how well they can cope with it.

Sometimes there is overt depression in the family: the patient may become depressed by the losses and difficulties in rebuilding life; relatives may become depressed by the burden of care, isolation and the feeling that no one understands. In elderly carers there is an inevitable worry about the future: "Who will look after him when I am gone?" Siblings may worry about how problems will affect them. There may be general anxiety and confusion about what has happened and what the future will hold. All relatives are likely to feel stigmatised and isolated.

Normalising emotional responses

The important thing to emphasise to the family during a session is the normality of any of these emotions, especially the negative ones. The feelings that families have, however intense, are typical of any family having to face the change and upset that can accompany living with schizophrenia. They may even be helpful in forcing family members to acknowledge that there are problems and thus to engage in treatment sessions.

Clinical example
This is an example of the therapist normalising the relatives' feeling of upset at the patient's disturbed behaviour.
M. Sometimes he comes to you and says "I want to do this." I say "Oh yes, of course. Why not?" Then he goes away and comes back and says "No, I changed my mind."
F. Yes, he changes his mind quick. So we can't ask him to go on holiday. He says "Yes" and then says "No, I don't want to go." We want to take him on holiday, but when he does things like that, we worry. We spend money and then he tells you no.
T. All that changing his mind, that's a very common problem. It's what relatives often experience with people with schizophrenia.

Therapists must allow relatives to admit to these feelings and not be taken aback or feel shocked by them. Negative emotions exist and should be acknowledged and listened to. However, what must also be done is to make sure that, during a session, negative feelings are not used as a way of attacking other family members. Overtly hostile, critical or intrusive statements need to be noticed by therapists and prevented from causing further argument and upset.

Positive reframing

One of the major aims of an intervention is to reduce relatives' expression of criticism. Criticism is fuelled by anger with the patient, which often stems from a misunderstanding of the patient's behaviour. We have found that the majority (70%) of critical comments are about the negative symptoms of schizophrenia. Relatives may not appreciate that these are part of the illness. Instead, they view them as being under the patient's control and consequently blame the patient for behaving badly. Part of the education programme is aimed at changing critical relatives' understanding of negative symptoms. Other components, particularly the problem-solving approach, are intended to help the patient overcome the negative symptoms. In the long term, these techniques are effective in softening relatives' critical attitudes. However, when criticism is expressed during a session, therapists should take immediate action to moderate its negative effect. The way to do this is called positive reframing. This is an important technique that therapists need to become familiar with and be able to practise as part of their training. It channels negative emotion so that it can be used constructively during a family session.

Positive reframing is a way of getting underneath negative emotion and pointing out that there is a positive reason for the intensity of the feeling. If relatives were not concerned and did not care, they would not be in a session trying to sort things out. We have always found it possible to find a positive aspect to even the most hostile or negative statement. This is an important part of being a therapist for these families.

For instance, rejecting remarks, such as "I can't stand living with you" can be reframed as the relative feeling so upset by the illness and what it does that he/she wishes that things were different. "I can't let you look after yourself" can be reframed as a worry that the person will not manage and might come to harm. "What will happen when I'm not here to look after you?" is a realistic worry about the future that both relative and patient need to consider. Following positive reframing, the relative should be encouraged to make a polite request for a change in behaviour.

Clinical example
This is an example of the therapist reframing the relative's criticism in terms of caring and then prompting the relative to make an appropriate request to the patient for a change in behaviour.
M.   She never washes her underwear.
T.   You really care about Emma's cleanliness.
M.   Of course I do.
T.   How would you like Emma to be?
M.   I would like her to wash her underwear regularly.
T.   Would you ask Emma that now?
M.   Emma, I would really like you to wash your underwear regularly.
This request can be followed by negotiation over how often Emma will try to perform the task in a week.

In this way it is possible to aim to increase coping skills so that the patient will be less vulnerable and more independent. Other strategies include not allowing family members to talk about someone else during a session. As discussed previously, making it a rule that relatives talk directly to each other means it is less easy to be overtly hostile, and is likely to defuse negative feelings.

Seeing family members separately

If negative feelings are prominent in a session, it may be necessary to see parts of the family separately for a while, in order to allow and acknowledge the intensity of emotional upset. Separate sessions for parts of the family can reinforce generational boundaries, cement marital alliances and allow therapists to listen to emotional issues without the worry that such topics will upset a patient or other family members. It may also be a useful way to engage families who feel that no one has previously listened to them or taken their problems seriously. However, even if some sessions are with separate family members, it can be helpful to bring the family back together for the last few minutes of a session and mention the issues that were brought up, if they involve the rest of the family. Unless the aim of a session is to separate hostile or intractable relatives (which will happen only in extreme cases), acknowledging and looking at areas of mutual concern is the beginning of the therapeutic process.

The use of relatives' groups and role play

If it is available, a relatives' group can be another helpful way of dealing with emotional issues (see Chapters 24 and 25). All the relatives will have felt the intensity of the feelings. The normality of such emotions can be demonstrated, feelings can be ventilated without fear of upsetting the patient, and families who have felt upset but have coped with it can discuss how this was done.

Very occasionally, if therapists are really stuck, role play can be used in a family or relatives' group. This is a powerful technique and has to be used with safeguards. Putting a critical or hostile parent into the role of the patient and asking the patient to demonstrate a relative's viewpoint, forces a relative to empathise with the patient's experiences. We have used this technique, but relatives and patient must be 'de-roled', therapists must take control and do it for a short time only, and any feelings and worries must be discussed carefully afterwards.

Summary

Emotional responses in families include guilt, loss, anger, depression and stigma. Therapists must be able to cope with these and help to normalise them. Many of the negative emotions fuel criticism by family members. Overtly negative statements during family sessions should be interrupted, and therapists need to be able to reframe them positively.

CHAPTER 10

How families affect professionals

The spread of conflict

There are strong emotional tensions in high-EE families. It is easy for them to be transmitted to the therapists and mirrored by them. If there are two parents, it is common for there to be conflict between them about how to tackle the problems raised by the patient. A frequent pattern is for the mother to be overinvolved and the father to be critical. The mother then criticises the father for being too hard, while he criticises her for being too soft.

Clinical example
This illustrates contrasting attitudes by two parents, which can lead to conflict.
F.   You see we take two different approaches. See, she's got a very soft approach. She always has had. Well, I mean, mothers do, don't they? I think really Paul has been, I should say, a mother's boy. And he plays on it a little bit sometimes. But I've been the other way. I don't believe in molly-coddling. I say she's too soft and she says I'm too hard.

Conflict can also develop between a single parent and a patient, and, in marital homes, between the patient and partner. The warring family members do their best to win one or other of the therapists over to their side. It can happen that one therapist is more sympathetic to one of the sparring partners, while the co-therapist leans towards the other. This can readily lead to a split between the therapists, which will impair their working relationship. Therapists should therefore always be on the lookout for the development of tensions with their working partner. When they occur, the first thing to do is to examine how they might reflect tensions between family members. Once the source of them has been identified, they can be dealt with effectively.

Sometimes conflict within the family can spread beyond the co-therapists, to the wider clinical team. The situation is ripe for this to happen when there are already divisions within the team, for example between health and social services staff, or between hospital and community staff. It is of the highest importance to preserve good working relationships within the whole group of staff involved with the family, or they will be unable to offer effective help. Regular communication within the team about the therapeutic activities with the family can help to prevent conflict. Once it is apparent, however, it is essential to hold a meeting of all the staff concerned to locate the source of the conflict. While this may sometimes stem from interprofessional rivalries and tension, such conflict can originate from the family, and this source should always be considered.

Doom and gloom

At some stage in their life with a person with schizophrenia, most relatives become overwhelmed by a sense of hopelessness and despair. It seems to them that, despite their best efforts and the help of professionals, the patient is making no progress.

Clinical example
This is an example of the patient communicating hopelessness to the relative, who then expresses it to the therapist.
M. I don't think John is getting any better. He's getting a lot worse. I'm very worried. You know you can't help him. He's very depressed. He's always contemplating suicide.

Relatives may openly communicate these painful experiences to therapists, who can easily then become overwhelmed and even come to believe that there really is no hope and that nothing that will help.

It is important for the therapists to bring these feelings to their support group. Their peers need to remind them that these feelings come from the family, rather than originating in themselves, and that there is always something that can be done, however small, that might lead to an improvement. Once it is clear that the source is the family, the group can begin to 'brainstorm' the problems. The group can act as a valuable resource for generating new ideas and ways of tackling problems when the therapists get stuck. With the support of their group behind them, therapists can better sustain families through periods of hopelessness.

Guilt and anger

Other responses shown by relatives to lack of progress by the patient are guilt and anger. Guilty relatives tend to contact a large variety of professionals and services, attempting to get them all to act on the patient's behalf. They are sometimes successful in engaging a variety of people, who get involved because they begin to feel guilty that they are not doing enough for the patient. In this respect they mirror the guilt of the relative. The usual result is a number of professionals working at crosspurposes, which is not helpful for the patient or the family.

The remedy is to convene a meeting of all the individuals and agencies involved with the family and to confine active work to the minimum number required. Help relatives understand their sense of guilt and emphasise that they are doing the best possible for the patient by working together with the therapists. Attendance at a relatives' group can also reduce feelings of guilt when relatives realise that they are not struggling in isolation with unique problems, but share much in common with others.

Angry relatives tend to blame the staff and the services for the patient's slow progress. By doing so, they often alienate the staff and actually receive a worse service than if they had not complained. Such relatives need help from the therapists to appreciate why they are angry and to lower their expectations for the patient. They may also need assistance in improving their relationship with other members of staff, which is likely to involve the therapists acting as advocates on behalf of the family.

Summary

Strong emotions originating in the family are communicated to the therapists and the other members of staff and may impede the process of working with the family. In general, if therapists begin to have strong feelings about the family, such as guilt, anger or hopelessness, it is important to recognise that they are likely to be mirroring emotions in the family and to discuss them with the co-therapist and with the support group. Once their origin is recognised, the therapists will find it much easier to deal with them and to continue with useful work.

CHAPTER 11

Leaving

Family work is time limited and has to come to a halt at some point. Sessions are usually held every fortnight for the first six to nine months and once a month thereafter. Some families will have sorted out their main problems by nine months, while others need regular sessions for as long as three years. Therapists may decide that the time has come to leave the family, or a therapist may have to leave for professional reasons. Either way, the family needs plenty of warning (at least one month and preferably more) of the leaving date so as to prepare themselves and to work through the feelings aroused.

Therapists may experience feelings of guilt and responsibility at leaving families. These should be explored in the therapists' support group, which is an essential component in any service.

Establishing a lifeline

If the therapist is leaving while work remains to be done, a replacement therapist may be found, and should be introduced to the family before the familiar therapist leaves. For families with obviously long-term problems, it is advisable to assign a more senior therapist, to provide greater continuity, to avoid the inevitable disruptions that accompany leaving.

If the therapists have come to the end of their work, they need to leave the family with a telephone number to contact them or some other appropriate professional. This acts as a lifeline that, from our experience, families do not abuse, but use when they have genuine need. The therapists need to warn the family that there may be a recurrence of old problems or the appearance of new ones, and to tell them that they should not be surprised by this, because it is in the nature of schizophrenia. Relatives may find themselves able to cope with these problems themselves, but if not they should telephone.

During discussions about the process of leaving, the family may express feelings of anger and loss about being deserted. They may feel that since they will be caring for the patient for many years to come, they will continue to need the support of the therapists. Establishing the lifeline of a contact number is one way of dealing with this. However, throughout the sessions the aim is to help the family to identify their strengths and to gain confidence that they have the resources to deal with their problems. Thus from the very beginning the therapists will be working towards the goal of the family's independence from them.

Reviewing the family work

As the sessions draw to a close it is natural for the family and the therapists to review what changes have occurred. The therapists will usually be able to identify positive changes in relatives' attitudes and behaviour towards the patients and in the patient's level of activity. However, family members may find it difficult to acknowledge the changes. Any alteration in the way they relate to each other can be seen as threatening, involving a leap into the unknown. The therapists may have to be content with their own recognition of the positive effects of their work with the family, without the additional satisfaction of the family's gratitude. Under no circumstances should they attempt to press the family to admit that change has taken place.

Rarely, one or more members of the family express the wish to stop the sessions before the therapists consider it is appropriate. This requires negotiation, particularly if family members disagree about it. However, it may lead to a premature ending of sessions. As above, the therapists should not attempt to prove to the family the value of their work together, as this will lead to confrontation and unproductive argument. The therapists have to accept that the family no longer want them to visit their home. Ways of responding to this are discussed in the final section of Chapter 23.

Summary

Families need plenty of warning of the therapists' intention to stop the sessions. Therapists should leave the family with a work telephone number on which they can be contacted. Changes that have occurred during the family work should be reviewed, but it may be difficult for family members to acknowledge them. Therapists are advised not to press this issue.

Part III

Emotional issues, problems of individuals and groups

CHAPTER 12

Anger, conflict, rejection

Despite what has been said earlier about dealing with emotional issues in general (Chapter 9), family members are likely to get angry with each other. Some families do not know how to discuss anything without having an argument. Sometimes just sitting in a room together will spark conflict in a family that has avoided issues or each other. Sometimes views are held so strongly, or feelings are so intense, that family members say hurtful and rejecting things to each other. At times these feelings may lead to violence – either verbal abuse, such as shouting, or physical abuse. Although it is unusual for the latter to happen during sessions, it can be part of the family interaction pattern. One of the commonest examples of this is when an overinvolved parent, usually a mother, is unable to put any limits on the behaviour of an adult son or daughter, who then can become overly demanding and threatening in the childish role or sick role he/she now occupies.

Defusing anger

Therapists must feel confident that they can defuse any anger and potential for actual violence. The social constraints of the family meeting may help. The expression of even very strong feelings may be tempered by having non-family members as witnesses. Rejecting or hurtful remarks can be defused by positively reframing them (see Chapter 9). Arguments and conflict can be defused by ensuring that each family member is listened to. If necessary, the rules of turn taking and listening can be formalised, by giving each family member, say, two minutes in which to make his/her views known. The other rules of family meetings will also help to defuse anger. For example, the rule about family members not talking about each other in the third person (e.g. "He is being difficult") but only directly to each other in the second person ("You are being difficult") is likely to lead to statements being toned down (e.g. to "I find that you can be difficult").

Another method of defusing angry statements is to ensure that individuals specify what it is that they are so cross about. Therapists must move statements from general (e.g. "You are so lazy") to behaviour (e.g. "I want you to get up in the morning"). Once behaviour has been specified, therapists and the family will have a problem to work on – something which can potentially be modified.

Clinical example

This illustrates the therapist asking the patient to focus on a specific problem instead of expressing general anger.

P.   I think it is outrageous. I mean somehow she's running. I know she's been in a car crash and she hasn't got much in her head, but really, just out of common decency, she wouldn't go out with somebody like that.

T.   It would help you, Colin, if we looked at what the problem's about, and just take it in turns to say what the problem is, so we can move towards a resolution.

Keeping control

Therapists should make sure that they keep control of the family if anger or potential violence is in evidence. Most families respond to clear and firm reminders of why they are meeting (to try to help with the problems) and of the rules outlined in Chapter 7. However, if repetitive argument develops, or if conflict seems to be escalating, it is important that therapists intervene. This requires skill and confidence, but it is a way of containing the fear that anger will generate and of making the family feel safe.

Clinical example

This is an example of the therapist intervening to prevent an angry exchange escalating further.

M.   It's been going on for a long time about the shirts. I say, "Full stop! Don't bring anything home at all. Get on with it."

P.   Bird brain, don't talk to me like that, and talk past me. You're a fool.

T.   David, it doesn't help very much if you make derogatory comments. If there's something that's upsetting you, we're here to try and help.

Some families may use the therapists' visits to enact their arguments, because of the safety that visitors imply. Therapists should make it clear that conflict and arguments are not tolerated and do not form part of a constructive family session. It can help to reframe the anger itself. This is done by talking about the strength of feeling that family members obviously have and how much it shows that they care about how difficult and upsetting things may be at present. This is a way of using the negative emotion constructively and helping the family to channel their strong feelings into making changes, rather than being destructive and feeling hopeless about the future.

Clinical example

This is an example of the therapist blocking the patient's criticism of his mother, reframing it positively and encouraging the patient to be constructive.

P.   The way she carries on with Edward – it's all wrong. It's not right at all. I'm saying that my mother's not strong enough to know that people can control her, quite easily control her, control her mind, but she's not strong enough to know that.

T.   It feels as if you're taking a lot of responsibility for what your mother does or for your mother's life in terms of whom she chooses. It seems that you're concerned about your mother's way of life.

P.   Well it is half concern for my mother, but the other half is things are rotten and going … [therapist interrupts].

T.   I was wondering whether you could say something different to your mother. If it's about concern, whether you can actually say what the concerns are about.

If, in extreme cases, families do not respond to any of the above, or if, for whatever reason, they stop listening to the therapists and shout or attack each other, then the therapists need to separate them, and each therapist should see part of the family system separately. Sometimes family members arrive at a meeting already angry and upset and this can make it difficult for therapists to start a constructive session. If family members are immediately seen separately, this enables both sides to calm down and the therapists have a chance to assess the problems and get difficulties reframed. If parts of the family are seen in this way it is still important to regroup for the last few minutes so that both sides can hear what has been discussed.

Model positive negotiation

Therapists must be able to deal with conflicts between themselves and to negotiate differences in a positive way. As described in Chapter 4, the therapists should show how a constructive resolution to genuine differences of opinion can be reached: this may be the only example a family is exposed to of how this can be done. Because of the role modelling they provide, therapists must also make sure that they do not 'take sides' with family members (unless in a planned way as an advocate), as this will leave others feeling neglected and misunderstood. Therapists need also to be aware that their own behaviour when under pressure, or when an argument starts, is important. The therapists should not shout back, nor should they show irritation or anger; neither should they make critical or rejecting remarks themselves, even if provoked. Remaining calm, talking in an even tone, not being visibly panicked or upset by a family's behaviour, and taking firm preventive action if necessary are important ways of ensuring safety and control. If therapists do encounter violence and hostility between family members, it will help to remember that the family will almost certainly have behaved in a much more extreme way at other times. Therapists are unlikely to elicit behaviour that is not already part of an established pattern. Even the most rejecting and angry remarks or actions will usually have been said or done many times previously; when they are demonstrated, therapists have an opportunity to allow the family to look at and begin to modify them.

If all the above tactics fail, therapists should try to stop everyone talking and to help all the family members to calm down. If possible, they could suggest that they will arrange another meeting in a few days, when everyone is a bit less upset. They should not arrange it there and then, but try to let the family know by telephone or letter when they would next like a meeting. If the family becomes angry with one or both of the therapists, and begins to shout or be threatening to them, the therapists will need to apologise, saying they did not mean to upset them but were there as arranged. If personal safety is being threatened, therapists should leave calmly and rapidly, and try to reconnect with the family later on that day or the next day to see if another meeting can be arranged, when, again, everyone is calmer.

Look at the positive aspects

Assuming that conflict or the threat of physical harm can be defused, therapists should aim to start looking at the problems that they illustrate. They should try to move the family away from negative escalation and begin to build in again positive aspects which family members have lost. We have found that even in very angry relationships, the fact that there is a relationship means that there is a positive side. Family members are likely still to care for each other and to want things to improve. Therapists can ask each family member to say something positive, to ask what they do like about each other. Occasionally family members fall silent at this point. Therapists can offer some suggestions about positive things that they have noticed. It may be that behaviour in the past has been positive but has not been tried recently. Positive behaviour can be neglected or taken for granted even in relationships not characterised by conflict; it needs to be elicited, valued and listened to, and therapists must help family members to do this for each other. If necessary, they should check that positive comments have been heard and registered – they could ask a family member to repeat the positive thing that has just been said about them.

Limit setting

If limit setting is a problem, the steps involved need to be gone through in detail. In a family unable to manage this, members need permission to set limits; they may then require a great deal of help both to set reasonable limits (agreed with the other person, not imposed) and to try them out consistently. This is discussed in detail in Chapter 13.

Unpacking a violent incident within the family

Finally, if actual violence has occurred, either before or within a session, the incident needs to be looked at in a further session in order to try to prevent it recurring. Some days after a violent event, when both sides are calm, therapists should go through the incident in detail. Both sides should give their version of events and should be listened to. Feelings which the violence caused should be elicited. Each side should tell the other what it felt like. Otherwise, it can be easy for one or both sides to pretend that the event was not that important. This loses the opportunity to feed back realistically how hurtful and upsetting it was to the victim, and how angry and upsetting it was to the perpetrator. Any triggering incidents should be clearly identified in order either to modify or to avoid them in future. Often a pattern will be obvious, and can then be interrupted.

Prevention

In order to try to prevent violence recurring, the family should try to rehearse ways of coping if a similar situation should arise. The perpetrator may be able to give warning of feeling angry (and possibly violent). Anger and conflict may be part of an impending relapse and help can then be organised for this. Simple strategies such as avoidance or calming down can be used. The angry person can be encouraged to withdraw to another room or go out for a walk for a while. How to call in help if things start to get out of control should also be discussed. Therapists should stress the need for family members to be able to feel safe. If necessary it may be possible to call in the care team, the general practitioner, or in extreme instances the police. Discussing these difficult options when everyone is calm is likely to help prevent dangerous outcomes in the future.

Summary

Anger and violence are frightening, but may form part of family interactions. Therapists need to defuse potentially escalating negative interchanges if at all possible. If necessary they should separate family members and see them separately. Therapists themselves must model positive interaction and settle differences by negotiation – they must not join in with family conflict. Once defused, negative patterns should be replaced by positive ones: often the family will need considerable help to do this. If violence has occurred within the family, it needs to be discussed calmly afterwards, and strategies for future prevention discussed and rehearsed.

CHAPTER 13

Dealing with overinvolvement

General considerations

It is important to recognise that overinvolvement usually has a much longer history than criticism, and consequently the time over which change can be achieved is also longer – years rather than months. It is not uncommon for a parent to describe overinvolved attitudes developing in the patient's childhood, sometimes in response to a serious physical illness in the child, to delayed milestones, or to some other deviation from normal development.

A crucial aspect of an overinvolved relationship is its symmetry. The relative and patient are equally dependent on each other and equally anxious about each other's welfare. The relative worries about how the patient would manage without her/him, and the patient shares the same anxiety owing to the lack of confidence that results from being overprotected.

Clinical example
This illustrates a patient's anxieties about the health of her overprotective mother.
M. I get it at night. I get woken up in the night. I'm having a lovely sleep and I get woken up. "Are you alright mummy? Oh, I thought you was dead."

It is necessary to deal with the anxieties of both partners in order to weaken the bond between them. Attempts to achieve separation rapidly and forcibly without dealing with the underlying emotional bonds often have the reverse effect, of pushing the partners closer together. One or other of them will almost invariably sabotage the arrangements made. Removing the patient from the home and placing him/her in staffed accommodation without working on the emotional issues around separation is likely to lead to the relative complaining about the quality of the care in the hostel or the patient slipping back home frequently.

Overinvolvement usually develops in a parent's relationship with a son or daughter. Only occasionally do we see it in other relationships, such as between partners. The point of trying to effect change in order to separate the overinvolved pair is that such a relationship not only overburdens the relative but also hinders a patient's recovery by preventing the practice of skills such as self-care. We work towards separation in order to allow the normal process of adult individuation to occur in the son or daughter and also to enable the patient to begin to contribute again within the family, thus alleviating guilt and feelings of uselessness.

In the case of partners, the aim is normally to encourage some recovery of the adult role in the family, even if this has been affected by the illness. For example, a patient who is a partner may not be able to manage a paid job but could still contribute by doing work around the house.

It is also important to aim for separation and independence in cases where a parent and son or daughter have become so locked together that the patient's demands cannot be refused. If the demands escalate, this situation can easily lead to resentment and violence, and can be dangerous. These issues are discussed in Chapter 12.

Relative's guilt

The emotion most often found to underlie overinvolved behaviour is guilt. Relatives may feel personally responsible for the patient falling ill and dedicate themselves to making everything come right for the patient. Thus they will attempt to do everything for the patient, which has the effect of undermining the patient's confidence and increasing dependence on the relative.

Clinical example
This illustrates a relative's sense of guilt at separating from the patient for a brief period to attend to her own needs.

W.   When I have left and been gone for a whole week, I'm worried sick in case he's overdone the pills or he's gone out and got himself drunk, and I'm saying "What if he's in the gutter somewhere?" It's my fault, you know. You get no peace. You can't go to the ends of the earth because they're here, and there's no way you can shut them out.

The relative's sense of guilt can be lessened by repeated assurance that relatives cannot cause schizophrenia. It can also be diminished by meeting others at a relatives' group. However, some relatives may find it a relief to talk about their guilty feelings one to one with the therapist.

Finding a lever

If the overinvolved relative and the patient are apparently satisfied with their relationship and there is no other adult in the household, it can be difficult for the therapists to find a lever to effect change. If another adult is present in the household then he/she may resent the closeness between the overinvolved couple, in which case he/she can be recruited as an ally by the therapists. Otherwise, a strategy we find useful with a single overinvolved parent is to draw his/her attention to the 'when I am gone' scenario. This is a common concern of elderly parents of adults with schizophrenia, who cannot see any prospect of another person or professional providing the same level of care after their death.

Clinical example

This is an example of a father presenting the 'when I am gone' scenario to the patient.

F.   I tell him every time I get a chance. I say, "Do something because later on if we die, I don't know who will look after you. While we live it's alright, but tomorrow you don't know."

The parent is asked to imagine what things will be like in, say, one year, five years and 15 years (the collapsed-time technique). This then becomes an argument for increasing the patient's independence and ability to care for him-/herself. In other families, patients may express discontent with the restriction on their freedom and the intrusion into their privacy. On the other hand, parents may resent the burden and the lack of privacy that the patient's dependence creates. Discontent in either partner provides an opening for the therapists to begin work.

Exploring anxieties about separation

In order to persuade patients and relatives to begin the process of separation, it is necessary first to explore the relatives' anxieties about what might happen if they relaxed their vigilance. They often protest that if they were to go out and leave the patient, the patient might damage the home or him-/herself. These fears of the worst outcome need to be discussed with the relative and the patient and their likelihood weighed up. They almost always turn out to be exaggerated.

Clinical example

This illustrates a mother's anxieties about allowing the patient to perform an age-appropriate activity.

M.   I don't like Cheryl going to the hospital by bus because she has to cross the road at the other end. At this end I can take her across the road myself.

T.   But isn't there a traffic light by the hospital?

M.   Yes, but she's always in another world. You can't trust her to look out for herself.

T.   Cheryl, is there a light to tell you when to cross, you know, with a green man on it?

P.   I think so.

T.   Do you think you use the light to help you cross safely?

P.   I think so.

The next example is of the therapist encouraging a mother to go on holiday and exploring her anxieties about leaving the patient.

Clinical example

T.   It sounds like you went away to friends before, for weekends and things.

M.   Yes, but since he's been ill, I don't.

T.   I wondered about that. Why's that?

M.   Probably just me. Just in case anything happens and they need me.

T.   What is your worst fear about what might happen while you're away?

M.   Er, just in case he got worse or, all sorts of things can happen, you know. All sorts of silly things, or in a sense they're not silly, are they? When you hear all these things that happen.

T.   But has anything like that ever happened that has made you worry?

M.   No, no, but it's within yourself and, oh, I don't know. I suppose sooner or later when you're a mother, you … I suppose you …

T.   I suppose there is always a possibility of those things happening. I mean, maybe you can't say they're not going to happen. But I suppose the likelihood is that they probably won't, and in a sense you do have to get on and live your life, and that's important.

It can also be useful to get relatives to face the impossibility of maintaining constant vigilance – they have to sleep at some time. We then negotiate with the relative to leave the patient alone on a trial basis for a short time, say half an hour. Of course, the therapists cannot guarantee that nothing disastrous will happen, but they can reassure the relative that the chances are very small indeed, and that it is a risk worth taking. The first small step is usually the most difficult and once achieved leads to more rapid progress.

In helping parents to choose an activity that will take them out of the home, there are a number of factors to consider. If there is a partner in the household, the two parents should be encouraged to go out together. Often the marriage has suffered because of the overinvolved parent's dedication to the patient and through conflict over the management of daily difficulties. The parents need to rediscover a sense of pleasure in each other's company and to experience some relief from the burden of constantly caring for the patient. They often seem to need the therapists' permission to relax and enjoy themselves. We formulate the permission as follows: "You have worked so hard to look after the patient that you have earned a rest". Relatives usually experience a considerable easing of the burden of responsibility when they find that they can leave the patient even for a short while without a tragedy occurring. During the relatives' brief absence patients should be set a task to perform which will increase their confidence and sense of achievement (see Achieving independence, this chapter).

Some relatives have no partner, in which case the therapists encourage the relative to resuscitate contacts with friends and relations outside the home. Often relatives have withdrawn from their social networks through shame and embarrassment, and have thereby lost a valuable source of emotional support.

Clinical example
This is an example of the therapist beginning to explore the possibility of a mother using her social network.
T.   Do you have any friends around here that are supportive for you, Sandra? Have you got any good friends around?
M.   What do you mean 'supportive'?
T.   Well, someone who will listen to you, who will support you in the same way that you support your niece and your son.
M.   Well, yes, I suppose so.

Relatives may also need encouragement to resume leisure interests they had previously, or even to return to work if they have given this up in order to look after the patient.

Overinvolved parents often have an additional fear of losing their relationship with the son or daughter once separation begins. We normalise this anxiety by pointing out that all children have to achieve psychological separation from their parents, although schizophrenia delays the process. Furthermore, once separation has been negotiated, the two partners have the opportunity to establish a new, more adult relationship. The parent may still need to come to terms with losing a child and can be helped with this by other parents in the relatives' group who have been through this process and appreciate the eventual advantages.

Replacing the role of carer

The person who takes on the role of carer often invests a great deal of emotion and energy in it, and it can become the sole source of satisfaction in their life. This has two main consequences for family work. First, informal carers may see the professionals as rivals, who are trying to oust them from their valued role. This rivalrous attitude can lead to carers becoming antagonistic to the therapists and criticising them for providing inadequate care. In this situation it is necessary for the therapists to congratulate carers on the excellent care they have been providing for the patient and to acknowledge that no one can adequately replace them. Nevertheless, for the patient to achieve independence, the carer has to gradually withdraw from the role. Second, the therapists have to help carers find an alternative role from which they can derive satisfaction. Voluntary activities for the mentally ill are one alternative, but may be too close to the role that is being relinquished. It is worth asking carers to remember what activities they enjoyed before the patient fell ill, and encourage them to build up one or more of those again.

Limit setting

One aspect of overinvolvement, excessive self-sacrifice, can be shown by relatives allowing the patient's disturbed behaviour to encroach too much on their own life. Alternatively, they may try to meet every demand the patient makes on them, however unreasonable, in the same way that some parents are overindulgent to their children. This behaviour stems from the relative's sense of guilt (see above).

In addition, relatives should be encouraged to respect their own needs and sense of comfort. This will inevitably involve them setting limits on the patient's behaviour and demands. On the other hand, patients should be given the opportunity to state what limits they would want the relative to observe with respect to overprotection and intrusiveness into their lives. In order to establish both these sets of limits, it is necessary to negotiate an agreement between the patient and relative. This needs to be based on mutual respect and should not be operated punitively: some relatives vacillate between no limits and unreasonable demands. Both partners to the agreement have to be prepared to maintain the limits firmly and consistently and not give in to persuasion, demands or threats. These can be difficult for relatives to withstand, particularly if they have a strong sense of guilt concerning the patient. If the relative appears incapable of maintaining firm limits, it is an indication for further exploration of guilty feelings. Relatives often benefit from permission from the therapists to establish limits. An example of limit setting by a relative is provided by a wife who told her husband she realised he could not help talking aloud to the voices but that he would have to do it in another room. An example of limit setting by a patient is that of a son who established with his mother that she could visit his flat only once a week instead of three times to check on his tidiness.

Some families are helped by formulating the limit as a contract, which both sides agree to and write down.

Achieving independence

While the parent is gradually letting go, patients need to build up confidence in their ability to look after themselves. The therapists seek agreement between family members on small achievable tasks for the patient to tackle. These have to be relatively undemanding at first, to minimise the risk of failure. Examples might be emptying the rubbish bin or washing underclothes once a week. It is a good plan to start with activities directed at self-care or care of the patient's bedroom, since these are often areas of intrusive concern by the overinvolved parent. A common response by the parent to the setting of such a task is to say that the patient does not do the job properly and it is better to take over.

Clinical example
This is an example of a wife with high standards finding it hard to tolerate the patient's less efficient ways of doing things.
T.   Michael, I was wondering if Polly asked you to do a task and she offered to help you, to work together with you to do it, would you feel more able to do the task?
P.   Yes.
T.   Have you ever told her this?
P.   No. Er, let's think now. Polly is like a back-seat driver. She has to have it done her way. That way doesn't suit me, so I down tools, you know. I down tools.
T.   I think it's very difficult when you've both got different standards for doing things. That must be difficult for you, Polly, particularly as you like things done to perfection.
W.   I probably set myself high standards, expecting them from everybody else too.
T.   Yes.
W.   That's about right, isn't it? I'm fussy.

The therapists need to work towards lowering relatives' expectations for patients' performance, and should therefore emphasise the impairments that linger for some time after an episode of schizophrenia. It is also necessary to point out that if the relative always takes over from the patient, the patient will never improve. These messages need to be reiterated many times before relatives' behaviour begins to change. Persistence is one of the greatest therapeutic virtues in this work.

In order to get the patient to spend more time away from a parent, therapists should help to establish links with people of the patient's generation. This is often impeded by the small social networks that patients sustain and by their lack of social skills. Sometimes a healthy sibling can be recruited as an ally to take the patient out and to introduce him/her to healthy young people. However, siblings may be understandably reluctant to bring their friends and the patient together, particularly if the latter is behaving oddly (see Chapter 20). Therapists can always fall back on introducing the patient to a day centre or drop-in centre, although a more 'healthy' environment is preferable. It is also helpful to find an interest that existed before the illness supervened and to encourage the patient to take it up again. Sometimes patients can be persuaded to join educational classes.

Strategic moves

During the course of family sessions we use a number of strategies directed at facilitating separation. These are used sparingly and with careful judgement as to the right moment to bring them into the session.

Changing seats

The therapists observe the seating arrangements in each session, as this is quite revealing of family relationships. Overinvolved relatives commonly sit next to patients and may make regular physical contact with them. A patient may be seated between the two parents, effectively separating them both physically and psychologically. At an appropriate juncture one of the two co-therapists will suggest changing seats with the parent or the patient. This can be introduced in an acceptable way, even in the home, by presenting it as an experiment that might improve communication. It is remarkable what a dramatic difference this physical separation can make to family interaction.

Splitting up the family

The therapists offer to see the patient separately from the relative. This emphasises that each person has different needs, and has personal issues that are appropriately kept private from the other person. If both parents are present in the household, the therapists will see them together to strengthen the marital alliance. If there is a healthy sibling available, the therapists may suggest that he/she is seen together with the patient, to facilitate peer bonding.

Recounting past separations

It can be helpful to ask overinvolved relatives to give an account of how they separated from their parents. This reminds the relative that such a move to independence is possible and desirable, and puts it in perspective as a normal stage in the development of every individual.

Paradoxical injunctions

When everything else has failed and we cannot think of any other means, we use a paradoxical injunction. We use this technique rarely because it works through the family members being unaware of what they are doing or why they are doing it. Furthermore, it enhances the therapists' power at the expense of the family's. In order to construct a bridge between the more usual approaches and a paradoxical injunction, the therapists can introduce it by saying, "It looks like our way of helping you hasn't worked. Let's try it your way – only more so." In the case of overinvolvement, we tell the relative and patient that they are not spending enough time together and that they must not let each other out of sight. The intention is that if they really follow this instruction they will get heartily sick of each other and begin to want some time apart. This intervention has worked when nothing else has been effective.

Summary

Overinvolved relationships are symmetrical and the anxieties and dependence of both partners need to be addressed. Brief trial separations should be negotiated as a way of tackling the anxieties. Relatives must be encouraged to attend to their own needs and to set limits to the patient's demands. The patient's confidence should be built up and he/she should be helped to establish social links outside the household. Strategic moves include changing seats during a session, seeing parts of the family separately and getting relatives to recount past separations.

CHAPTER 14

Grief

Grief and loss are common emotions families experience with long-term mental illnesses such as schizophrenia. There are two types of loss: loss of the person they used to know and loss of the hopes and aspirations they had for that person. It is in the nature of the illness that negative symptoms, such as lack of motivation, apathy and social withdrawal, often persist long after the acute phases of the illness have subsided. Hence child care, household responsibilities and employment are all too often affected. The patient may not provide any social company for the family. As a result, families may feel they have lost the person they used to know. Unfortunately, the illness often starts in adolescence or early adulthood, when the patient is at a critical stage in life and is expected to achieve most. Hence education, work and relationships are often disrupted. Consequently, families may feel they have lost all hopes and aspirations for the person. Moreover, their grief is compounded by the fact that, unlike grieving for a deceased person, patients are still alive, only they appear as strangers, many of the familiar aspects of the person having vanished.

Part of the therapists' job is to help families to overcome their grief. Enough rapport has to be developed to enable families to discuss their feelings. Some families may deny that there has been any loss or refuse to acknowledge any possibility of patients relapsing. Instead, their expectations for the patient's performance remain high. Sometimes patients share families' unrealistic expectations and keep trying to achieve well beyond their abilities, which causes frequent disappointment, stress and relapse. This can lead to a loss of confidence and a negative cycle of hopelessness for both patients and relatives. Some emotionally overinvolved relatives tend to refuse to talk about what the patient is like at the moment but hark back constantly to past good memories, when the patient was a child. With these families, the therapists' job is to lower their expectations by educating them about the effects of the illness. It may take several months to work through the family's denials.

The main task is to get families to acknowledge the reality of the loss without losing sight of the positive sides that still exist. Families can be encouraged to express their profound feelings of loss and devastation, which could be normalised by the therapists' sharing of their experience of families who have gone through similar stages.

Clinical example

Relatives' feelings of grief were discussed in this group and normalised.

Mrs A   I can't feel the same as I did. Too much has been taken out of me. If anything happened to him I'd be terribly upset, but I don't think it would hurt permanently.

Mrs B.   [Interrupts] It would have been a relief, dear. I felt this when Andrew was so ill I would rather he had died and I mean that. I didn't want the boy ill like that.

T.   It's not unusual to feel like that with these illnesses: it can make you very upset to see people change and then to have to cope with all the problems.

Patients should also be encouraged to share their own experiences of the illness to help their families to understand and empathise. At times it is advisable to do grief work about loss of the person in the relatives' group or separately, as it might be too painful for patients to hear. A relatives' group can be useful to share feelings and to demonstrate how some families might have seen some progress over time, despite their losses. Therapists should convey realistic hope and elicit the advantages of still having the person there. Once families can acknowledge their losses and see the positive attributes left, a structured behavioural strategy using graded tasks could be employed to maximise these positive attributes, as described in Chapter 8.

Summary

Grief is a common experience in the family when a member suffers from an illness that can be chronic and often disabling. In the case of schizophrenia, it could be grief for the loss of the person they used to know or grief for the loss of the hopes and aspirations for the person. It often is a combination of both. Relatives' groups are safe venues for relatives to express their grief openly, without the fear of upsetting patients, and to share their feelings. Therapists should encourage families to overcome their grief; to see the positive qualities that the patients still have; and to lower their expectations. Once families can acknowledge their losses and see the positive attributes that remain, small realistic goals can be set to enable progress.

CHAPTER 15

The vulnerability of adult patients

When people have had the problems associated with schizophrenia for some years, they may have residual disabilities, which have to be coped with. These can include positive symptoms, such as distressing voices or delusions, poor concentration, and also negative symptoms, such as apathy, low motivation and self-neglect. Distressing voices and delusional ideas sometimes respond to individual sessions (known as cognitive–behavioural therapy for psychosis). This can be suggested to patients and their families, and therapists should be able to advise about local availability.

Those who had an early onset of illness may always have been socially isolated. Even with a later onset, social networks tend to become restricted through the impairment of social skills by the illness, because social withdrawal is quite common and on account of the stigma of mental illness.

Clinical example
A mother described her daughter's clinging behaviour from an early age.
M. Elaine didn't like her father very much. It's always been me ever since she was born. She was a difficult baby. She screamed and didn't sleep very much as a child, and wherever I went Elaine had to go. Even when she was young, if I went into friends I was being called out again. You know, the others all played, but not Elaine, "Mum, come in!" It's always been the same with Elaine. Very, very pathetic.

For all of these reasons it may be true that patients are not as competent as they were before the illness; they may have lost skills and confidence, and lack experiences such as being able to live independently. Carers who live with such patients, particularly carers who are parents, may find it difficult to assess accurately the level of residual problems and to encourage and allow social functioning to recover. This is often part of overinvolvement, in that a parent may not accept adult functioning in the patient and may continue to treat her/him as a child. This is discussed in Chapter 13.

However, it can also happen that carers perceive accurately that patients are not able to cope with various problems. Therapists need to achieve a balance between encouraging as much independence as possible and acknowledging with the patient and relatives that there are problems that will continue to need help from carers. At best, patients can be encouraged to specify and ask for this help, and over time the level can be reduced. In other cases patients are not allowed even to try things for themselves and in this pattern patients themselves may see no need to change anything – they may be perfectly comfortable with the status quo.

Sexuality

An area where the issue of actual dependence versus fears of vulnerability is highlighted is that of sexuality. Parents, particularly of adult daughters, may find it extremely difficult to cope with the fact that the patient is likely to have sexual needs and, further, many choose as partners people who would not previously have been welcomed by the family unit. In long-established illness, partners are likely to be other patients, who may have as many problems as (or even more than) the patient. Another pattern is for sexual contacts to be casual rather than permanent, as intense relationships may be difficult to manage. Unprotected sexual contacts carry the risk of sexually transmitted disease, including AIDS, and also of pregnancy. Both of these raise understandable fears in carers.

Therapists should aim to allow for a realistic and frank discussion of sexual needs in adult patients. It is not an issue for all patients as for some social withdrawal and their own reticence will preclude it. However, for others it may be the first chance they have had to discuss it at all with their relatives. All the antipsychotic drugs in common use can interfere with sexual function in both men and women. Yet these side-effects are rarely enquired about by professionals and patients may be reluctant to mention them. Sexuality needs privacy and acceptance by the rest of the family. Ways of achieving this may have to be discussed. The fears families may have about the risk of disease and pregnancy should be brought into the open. Often patients have taken responsibility for themselves, but may not have mentioned it, or are not believed; this should be clarified. Usually families' worst fears are not realistic and the likelihood of various negative outcomes should be looked at and reappraised.

Pregnancy raises particular worries, including the possibility of whether the baby will inherit problems, whether the patient will be able to look after a baby or whether carers will have to take on yet another job and whether the patient should have the baby at all. Again, these need to be brought out and the family encouraged to discuss the options and come to some agreement. Usually the patient is the best person to set out the terms of such an agreement and by encouraging this therapists reinforce the responsible and adult side of a patient's behaviour.

Some families may refuse to talk about sexuality. It may be felt to be too painful, it may be culturally unacceptable or it may be seen as inappropriate. Any problems will be denied. It is not necessary to insist that a family faces these issues, but if it is an area where the family identifies problems then therapists should help to facilitate solutions.

Social competence

Another area of vulnerability may be social competence. Can a patient manage the usual problems that many adults have to deal with – managing money, street crime, coping with more competent friends, not being exploited by others?

Clinical example
This illustrates a mother's anxieties about her son's ability to budget.

T. So what are the things that James already has going for him? He can prepare his own meals?

M. Oh yes. He prepares them alright. Gets his clothes in the washing machine. He can iron. Well, he's ironing because he was at cubs. You should see these uniforms: he does them beautiful. That part's alright, but the money part. To save. If he got fifty pounds, he'd go out there tonight and spend the fifty pounds. And I think it's because he knows he can come and live here. Whereas if someone was going to say, "Where's my rent?" or "I take it away from you", they'd be more responsible.

T. So you have some fears about his not being able to budget.

There may be particular (and possibly valid) fears that patients will be mugged when going down the street or that they cannot manage things like bus rides or trips out; sometimes even crossing the road is felt to be too risky. Again, as in overinvolvement, the reality and likelihood of a negative outcome should be discussed and fears of a 'disaster' looked at calmly. The patient's views, while not always realistic, should be taken seriously and therapists should try to use patients as the agent of change whenever possible. As usual, fears should be narrowed down from the general ("He might get run over") to the specific ("How can we help him to get used to crossing roads?") and then the real problems, if they exist, can gradually be worked on.

The aim of the therapist with these issues is to encourage realistic but achievable aims which help a patient begin to function as an adult again, despite any residual problems. While this may not be possible to achieve in all areas of functioning (long-term patients may always need help with some aspects of daily living), often there are islands of competence, and these need to be noted and developed.

Summary

Many families have to help patients cope with residual disabilities. It can be difficult for relatives to assess these accurately and to help patients recover as much independence and adult functioning as possible. Two particularly difficult areas are the sexual needs of patients and their social competence. Therapists need to encourage families to focus on these problems and aim at achievable solutions.

Stigma

Society by and large still has a stereotyped view of the mentally ill. In the case of schizophrenia, the beliefs that these patients are violent, show sexually inappropriate behaviour and suffer from split personality still prevail. This is further complicated by the unpredictability of the illness. Some sufferers may relapse quite suddenly and the cause of the relapse may not always be clear. Some chronic sufferers may be stigmatised because they display the obvious residual negative symptoms of self-neglect, lack of motivation, social withdrawal and odd or bizarre behaviour. Rigidity or tremor as side-effects of major tranquillisers may also lead to stigmatisation. Sometimes the sufferer's sense of being stigmatised may be based on past disturbed behaviour which was socially unacceptable. Furthermore, there is still often an assumption that families may have caused schizophrenia in some way. Some families, particularly Asian families, may believe that if the offspring suffers from a major mental illness the whole family has failed or 'lost face'. It is still common in Western culture for parents to believe that they must have failed to some extent in bringing up the child for him/her to suffer from schizophrenia.

As a result, families and patients may feel rejection, real or perceived, by relatives, friends and society as a whole. The sense of rejection is often mixed with feelings of guilt, anger, inadequacy and hopelessness. Sometimes families tell only close relatives or friends about the illness. If patients have been admitted to a psychiatric hospital or psychiatric ward, some families ensure that nobody outside the family knows about it. Because of the sense of failure and fear of not being accepted by others, families often isolate themselves. They avoid contact with people who they fear might look down on them. Healthy siblings in the household often distance themselves from the family as far as possible through shame and embarrassment (see Chapter 20). Some families even go to the extreme of moving to a new neighbourhood in order to conceal the fact that their relative has had a major nervous breakdown.

Intervention

It is important to explore the sense of stigmatisation and isolation with families. Sometimes families may not say that they feel stigmatised but behave as if they were by isolating themselves from larger networks, from which they could receive support and social company. Education helps to demystify the illness and get rid of the guilty feeling that it is the families who cause the illness. It also helps to normalise families' feelings. However, the two initial education sessions are often not enough and therapists may have explicitly to relate information on a specific family problem or to how they construe the illness. Relatives' groups are often a good arena for relatives to share and normalise their feelings, grievances and past experiences.

Clinical example

This example is taken from an interchange in a relatives' group.

Mrs M.   I can't have Elaine with other relatives because they get very irritable. They don't understand Elaine and even shoot questions at her. They think that pushing her # is helping her, which it isn't.

Mrs T.   I'm very sensitive to the fact that our visitors would perhaps put Robin on edge and set him back. I find that I'm embarrassed a little bit because my relatives have to sort of make allowances for Robin.

Mrs M.   We all want our children to be better and to behave normal and be like us. But all the time we're aware that they're ill and we're making up excuses, really, either for ourselves or for others, for people not to notice that our children are ill.

Mrs T.   You can't treat people like that! They would know, and you embarrass them by trying to do it.

Relatives in a later group discuss the stigma of mental illness and the need to explain to the neighbours.

Mrs A.   I don't hide the facts.

Mrs B.   I carry on as normally as possible.

T.   What do you tell people?

Mr B.   That Peter is sick and had a breakdown, had schizophrenia.

Mrs B.   But people don't know what you're talking about with schizophrenia.

Mr B.   Nervous breakdown seems to be accepted. But the trouble is there is nothing wrong with him – he's a fine-looking chap.

Mrs A.   I think you have to let other people know what's wrong with them. You have to explain if they don't know about it. I told a friend at work and they were quite sympathetic.

More sensitive issues, such as child abuse, or problems that are uncommon to the rest of the group, such as an offspring or a sibling being the sole carer, may not be discussed. Therapists need to be alert and sensitive to these issues and to deal with them within the individual family setting.

To help patients break out of isolation, therapists need to be sensitive as well as persevering. Patients may have had years of isolation, as a result of which they are likely to lack confidence in their social competence. They may be easily embarrassed or intimidated. They may fear that they will be rejected because they have had the experience of a mental breakdown. Their fear may also come from past experiences of psychotic symptoms causing social embarrassment. Thus therapists should be empathic but encourage realistic expectations. Going through the advantages and disadvantages of continuing to isolate oneself from a larger network might help. Patients should be persuaded that the occasional symptom does not necessarily impede their ability to socialise. However, with some patients there might be a genuine lack of social skills rather than a lack of motivation. In these cases therapists should encourage the patient to practise socially relevant tasks. Graded tasks and task assignments as experiments can help to persuade patients to go out and mix more. Therapists or family members may have to accompany patients on the first couple of outings.

Furthermore, therapists need to persuade patients to talk to the appropriate people in the right context about their experience of mental illness without feeling shame. The idea is that patients should have the choice of telling people about their experience or not, without feeling that the experience is so shaming that they have to conceal it under all circumstances. To do so would negate any opportunity for support from any informal network.

Helping carers to form relationships outside the immediate family is an important aspect of family work if isolation is a problem. At times it is difficult to tease out whether isolation results from a sense of stigmatisation or from overinvolvement. However, families often cope better if there is a larger network from which they can ask for help or find relief. The usual excuses for not going out are "I'm too tired", "I haven't got enough time", "My son needs me" or "He can't be left on his own". There may be an element of truth in this, but it is important for therapists to push so that families can break out of their isolation. It often helps to improve the quality of their relationships, reduce the burden on relatives, reduce overinvolvement and reinforce generational boundaries. Sometimes it is useful to frame it as "Everyone in the family needs to look after themselves in order to cope". Hence neither patients nor relatives are singled out. In some very entrenched families, therapists may have to frame it in altruistic terms, such as "You need to look after yourself to help the patient" or "The patient needs to be on her own to promote independent functioning".

Just as with patients, relatives need to be persuaded to test their beliefs that people would reject or look down on them because they care for someone with schizophrenia. Cognitive–behavioural techniques of gentle persuasion to undertake short outings to test out their fears and then gradually to increase the difficulty of tasks apply equally to relatives and patients.

Summary

Many families feel stigmatised and isolated. As a result, they often avoid contact with people from whom they could receive support and social company. Helping carers and patients to break out of their isolation is an important aspect of family work. Sometimes it is difficult to tease out whether carers do not go out because of emotional overinvolvement or fear of rejection. Therapists need to enquire explicitly and deal with the cause accordingly. Some patients lack social skills or confidence because of the chronicity of their illness. A cognitive–behavioural technique of setting graded realistic tasks is useful to test out their beliefs of being looked down upon and to encourage both carers and patients to venture out.

CHAPTER 17

Absent family members

How to get everyone in the family involved

As discussed in Chapter 2, the recruitment of families should be attempted at a time of crisis, when they are likely to feel most in need of professional help. Most families first come into contact with services after a period of disturbance at home, during which virtually everyone in the family will have been affected by the patient's disturbed behaviour. The practice of beginning family work with education also helps to get every family member involved. Therapists should send families the message that it is important for all members to be present so that everyone has some understanding of what the illness is. During the education sessions, there should be a strong message that every family member can help by creating a supportive and encouraging environment to prevent relapse. It should be emphasised that:

(a) the family is not sick and hence is not being treated;
(b) therapists are there to deal with some of the problems the family is likely to have as a result of having a relative suffering from schizophrenia;
(c) relatives are valuable assets and allies of the professionals in helping patients.

In this way, the logic of getting everyone actively involved is made clear. The emphasis on a positive approach and collaboration during therapy also helps to engage family members. Therapists should be sensitive to a particular family's needs and identify and emphasise its strengths. Time should be spent listening to the family's experience and the involvement of each individual member so that the family feel they are listened to and understood. Similarly, family members' past attempts to cope should be listened to and respected as their best effort, no matter how undesirable these might seem to therapists. In order to establish alliances with individual members, therapists should understand the ongoing family issues as well as the demands on and problems of each family member. Hence it is quite a demanding task to establish rapport with each family member, as well as with the family as an entity. Moreover, therapy goals and tasks should be set only after each family member's view has been sought and any disagreements resolved.

Involving the 'peripheral' family network for support

The definition of 'family' varies across cultures. Relatives who are counted as peripheral family members by many white people in Britain may be seen by others as close family members who should be actively involved in family matters. In any culture, if there is a family crisis, distant relatives may rally round quickly to help out. Hence they are often useful resources for the family. While this may be particularly true for families who have immigrated to Britain, questions should always be asked about the peripheral family as a potential source of support.

Clinical example

T.   Do you have any relatives that you can ask for help?
Mrs A. Well yes I suppose I do have my cousin in Croydon. I can go and see her for a break, or get on the phone.

Regardless of culture, different people may be included within the term 'family'. Hence therapists should be sensitive to this issue and enquire who is around and involved in helping patients. Sometimes the important people are identified in the course of discussing a family's past attempts to cope. Important people in the network should be invited to family meetings even though they are not close relatives.

Coping with non-attendance

Non-attendance of family members cannot be ignored and should be dealt with as it occurs. Therapists must give the clear message that everyone is important and their active involvement is needed to help patients. Relatives may be out during the time of the meeting, or sometimes hover around in the next room, making their presence known but not coming into the meeting. In either case they should be invited to join the meetings.

It is not uncommon for the father of a patient to opt out of family meetings, particularly if the mother has shouldered the main burden of care. Fathers often give the excuse that they cannot take time off work. Therapists should schedule at least one meeting outside working hours to accommodate working parents. It is easy to ignore an absent father but this is a tactical mistake since his absence is often a statement in itself of a lack of involvement in the caring role, and exerts a powerful influence on the family.

Relatives may not attend family sessions for a variety of reasons. It could be that the person concerned has missed a meeting and the date of the following meeting is not passed on. This often reflects overinvolved relatives' attitudes that they can deal with patients' problems best on their own. They may feel that there is no need to involve other family members, hence dates of future meetings are not conveyed to them. The simplest way to deal with this is for therapists to say that they understand that there is a lot going on for the family and perhaps it is difficult for them at the moment to organise everyone to be there. Therapists can offer to write to each member individually for a limited time to establish regular attendance.

Non-attendance may also be a reflection on the therapeutic relationship if the individuals concerned feel they have been poorly understood or attacked unfairly in previous meetings. Or it may be that the absent members do not appreciate their role in helping the patient or that they simply do not understand or value the help being offered. Regular feedback from relatives, both verbal and written, helps to alert therapists to these problems.

If there is a problem with the therapeutic relationship, the person's feelings should be accepted and validated. Therapists should make clear the intentions behind what they did in previous sessions and could even acknowledge that their actions unfortunately may not have had the desired effect. Most people will respond positively to this type of genuine and open approach.

If the reason for non-attendance is not seeing the value of family meetings or personal involvement, the rationale should be reiterated and any concerns or worries worked through. Sometimes, relatives do not attend meetings because of their fear of change. The fear could be based on the experience that patients relapse during times of change. Therapists should reassure them that gradual change is often productive and does not necessarily lead to relapse, particularly if there is a supportive environment.

Another type of fear is that overinvolved relatives are often not sure what their life would be like if the patient became more independent. This can be dealt with as described in Chapter 13.

Lastly, relatives sometimes continue to be absent despite a lot of effort to get them to attend. Realistically, therapists have no option but to persevere with parts of the family. Often the non-attenders eventually come through curiosity or because they find they are affected by these meetings as a result of changes in other members. If members refuse to attend despite being asked repeatedly to do so, this may have to be accepted eventually. Whatever the reasons may be for non-attendance, if the members concerned do start to attend meetings, therapists should be warm and welcoming. Their efforts in attending meetings should be appreciated.

Therapists should not necessarily accept any excuses for non-attendance at face value. Often, non-attendance is connected with other important family issues which those concerned do not want to reveal and these possibilities should be considered.

Coping with lack of interest in meetings

Sometimes relatives come to meetings and yet show a distinct lack of interest. They can be silent all through meetings and be reluctant to express their opinions even when asked. At the extreme, some relatives doze off or read the newspaper during family meetings. At other times, family members, particularly the patient, may wish to leave in the middle of the meeting. If this happens, an attempt should always be made to ask them to return. This is preferably done by another family member, but if this is not possible one of the therapists should ask them to return. This emphasises that their presence is important in the meeting even if they refuse to come back.

Non-verbal messages like leaving the meeting or reading the newspaper should be explored and clarified. The message could be that they felt misunderstood or undervalued or that they simply did not understand the help being offered and what is expected of them. These could be dealt with as outlined above. In particular, one of the therapists present at the meeting should try to form an alliance with the disaffected member, regularly asking his/her opinion and requesting feedback. Should therapists allow such a lack of interest to persist, relatives may exaggerate their behaviour in order to get their message across, do something else to sabotage the therapists' efforts to help, or simply stop attending family meetings altogether.

Summary

Engagement is often helped by the message that therapists are not there to treat the family but to deal with some of the problems the family may have as a result of a member suffering from schizophrenia. Relatives should be seen as assets and allies of the professional to help patients. The definition of 'family' can be quite loose; important but distant relatives should be identified and be included in meetings. Non-attendance of family members should be treated seriously and therapists should try their best to make sure that every family member attends regularly. Similarly, lack of interest during family meetings should be explored and the message dealt with accordingly.

CHAPTER 18

Helping marital families

Although many of the problems that arise in marital households are the same as in parental households, there are also some important differences that need to be considered. Partners can be just as critical as parents but are much less likely to be overinvolved. On the rare occasions when overinvolvement is found in partners, they have often adopted a parenting role in respect to the patient.

Task sharing

As with parents, criticism from a partner is usually directed at the patient's negative symptoms. If the patient is inactive, this has an effect on the household economy, and shifts the whole burden of wage earning and housekeeping onto the partner. In addition, there may of course be the responsibilities of child care, and statutory and non-statutory agencies (e.g. social services, child guidance, nursery care, after-school facilities) may need to be involved if this becomes problematic. Sometimes other relatives, such as the partner's or patient's parents, may be available to help. It can then happen that the patient is left without a contributory role in the family, which in itself is demoralising. In approaching this problem it is important to encourage the family members to be as flexible as possible. Reversal of 'conventional' roles may be a solution with a male patient: the wife going out to work while the husband cares for the home or children, or both. If this is not possible, it is helpful to negotiate which specific tasks he should undertake, such as decorating a room, mending or fixing things, or doing shopping.

Clinical example
In this session, the therapists help a husband and wife negotiate a task.
T.   So, Amos, you've said that it would be helpful if you'd be more able to do the task that Amy asked you to do, if she assists you with it.
P.   Yeah, sometimes.
T.   Amy how do you feel about that, about helping him?
W.   I don't mind, no.

T.   How would you feel about it, though, if Amos was to mow the lawn for you despite the fact you have different ways of doing it?

W.   Oh, it don't matter how you cut the grass really, does it? It would just be nice if he did it.

For any patient, help may be required with improving skills in shopping, budgeting and cooking. It is important for therapists to distinguish between the lack of opportunity to exercise a skill, as can happen with an overprotective relative, and a basic lack of the necessary skill. In the former case, work with the family is indicated. In the latter case, the therapists should consider referral of the patient to an occupational therapy department, day centre or local education classes. As always, the healthy partner should be encouraged to notice and praise the patient for successfully completing small tasks.

In the unusual situation that the partner is overinvolved, he/she will need to be persuaded to give up some of the responsibility shouldered for the patient. The approach is the same as with overinvolved parents, namely to explore the relative's anxieties about the possible dangers of giving the patient more scope, to give the relative permission to offload some of the responsibility, and to encourage partners to try out a small shift in the balance of responsibility. Pressure from other relatives in a relatives' group can be a potent force for producing change in this area.

Loss of a confidante

A warm and mutually supportive relationship is the basis for a good marriage. Schizophrenia can erode this basis by impairing the patient's emotional responsiveness to a partner and the patient's ability to provide support. The partner may find it difficult to accept that the loss of what they valued in the marriage is a result of the illness and not a deliberate withholding by the patient. It is not uncommon to find a high-EE partner harbouring a deep sense of disappointment and even bitterness.

Research has shown that depression is associated with the lack of a confiding relationship. If schizophrenia makes it impossible for the patient to fulfil this role, the partner should be encouraged to find someone else who can act as a confidante. Some confidantes may make the patient jealous and genuinely threaten the relationship with the partner, so the emphasis is on finding a friend, not an alternative relationship. Partners may find an appropriate confidante through a relatives' group or other supportive meetings (such as those run by MIND or the National Schizophrenia Fellowship).

Re-establishing a warm relationship

We have generally found that if relatives' critical attitudes can be moderated, warmth towards the patient returns spontaneously. In the case of parents this is a consequence of the natural investment of positive emotions in their child. In marital partners, however, the warmth would have had to be present in the relationship at the beginning if it is to re-emerge. If the marital relationship was not particularly good to start with, the best one can hope to achieve is the sharing of tasks in a neutral atmosphere. If the relationship was initially warm, it might still require a special effort to resuscitate it. Three main strategies can be employed:

(a) Ask each partner to say something positive about the other. If they complain that they cannot think of anything positive in the current relationship, then ask them to remember a positive aspect of the person in the past.

(b) Ask each partner to say something they would like the other person to do for them and negotiate for this to be carried out. Make sure that the task is well within the person's capabilities. Even a simple activity such as making a cup of tea for the other person can shift the relationship in a more positive direction.

(c) Find something that the partners would enjoy doing together outside the home and set them the task of trying it. As before, if they assert that there is nothing at present that they enjoy together, ask them to review the history of their relationship to find a suitable activity.

Sexuality

Both the patient and partner may be reluctant to raise the issue of their sexual relationship, but it is important for the therapists to introduce it tactfully. Schizophrenia itself can diminish libido, but so can neuroleptic drugs, including the new atypical antipsychotic medications. In men these can inhibit erection and ejaculation. If any of these problems exist, the possible causes should be presented to the partners and the patient's medication should be reviewed. A diminution in a partner's sexual interest and activity may be interpreted as a sign of loss of love and affection. It is therefore important that the alternative explanations be discussed.

If alterations in the drug regime are not helpful or not possible and the partners want further help with their sexual relationship, referral to a therapist specialising in sexual problems is indicated.

Clinical example
Relationships can often suffer after a long illness. This was discussed in some detail in one group meeting, where a wife found her husband's renewed sexual interest in her very difficult to cope with.

T.   There's a point here about giving support. You don't want to give support Mrs A and you two [Mr and Mrs B] find you are arguing about the amount of support John [son] needs.

Mrs A.   But there's a lot of feeling between you two [Mr and Mrs B]. Hugh idolises me and I don't hate the sight of him, but as far as being a husband and wife goes there's a lot been killed off, and I feel at times as if I've been cut into little pieces and they've all got a piece each and I'm just not me...

T.   Did you [Mrs D] find it a problem when your husband was out of hospital?

Mrs D.   Yes, it was at first.

T. Did you find that the relationship built up again?

Mrs D. No, not quite. It got better but it took a long time.

Mrs A. He came to meet me the other night. It sounds nice but I can't even walk home on my own any more.

T. It sounds as if you've got used to managing things by yourself.

Mrs A. I have. After all this time, it's a weird feeling that Hugh can even feel this way.

Mrs D. It sounds like a good sign.

Mrs A. It's a good sign for him getting better but its a terrifying sign for me if I can't put back what he wants, and I don't really think I can. I would be his best friend, but if he wants more than that I don't really think I can cope with it.

T. Have you said to him that you might build up the relationship gradually? Do you think it might be easier if you took it in stages?

Separation

In parental households, one of the major aims is to increase the independence of patients, with the possible result that they set up a household of their own. We would not start out with the aim of separating partners, although this outcome is usually raised by one or both partners during the course of work with them. Sometimes, despite the best efforts of the therapists, the partners remain irreconcilable. Under these circumstances it is desirable for the therapists to help them to separate in as constructive a manner as possible. This will usually involve assisting the partner to express guilt about deserting the patient and exploring anxieties about the possible disastrous outcomes, such as suicide or vagrancy. Partners rarely have the same degree of commitment to patients as parents do, so that if they separate, the partner is unlikely to provide much ongoing support for the patient. Possible alternative sources of emotional and practical support for patients need to be identified and brought into the picture, so that they are not left completely isolated.

If there are children in the household, their welfare takes precedence, and social services must be involved (see Chapter 19).

Summary

There are some specific problems that arise in marital households. These include sharing the burdens of wage earning, housekeeping and child care, the partner's loss of a confidante, and the effects of the illness and its drug treatment on the couple's sexual relationship. Therapists need to work towards re-establishing a warm relationship between the partners. Occasionally their task is to help the couple separate as painlessly as possible. If there are partners in a group, it can be a safe place in which to discuss marital difficulties.

CHAPTER 19

Children in the household

The children of a parent with schizophrenia may be adults, in which case they often take on some of the roles of carers. This is discussed in Chapter 20. However, if they are under the age of 16, there are a number of issues concerning their emotional development that need to be considered by the therapists. If there are young children in the household, social services are quite likely to be involved, or they may need to become involved. Hence the therapists should be prepared to develop a close liaison with social services.

Some 40 years ago it was relatively rare to find young children in a household with a parent suffering from schizophrenia. With the implementation of community care, this situation is becoming more common.

Timing of parents' marriage

The most usual circumstance is that the parents married when they were both well and that one of them subsequently developed schizophrenia. Any children are therefore likely to have experienced normal parenting for a period before the onset of the illness. Their response to the illness will depend, of course, on their age at the time, but also on the way in which the other parent responds to it. The onset of schizophrenia often creates anxiety and confusion in the marital partner, who may, as a result, be unable to help the children deal with their own emotions. Therefore it may be necessary for the therapists to spend time with the children, encouraging them to express their understanding of their parent's illness and their responses to it.

If the parents married when one was already ill, the well parent may have known what he/she was taking on and would have been able to explain it to the children when they reached an appropriate age. On the other hand, the children will never have experienced continuous normal parenting from one of their parents and may have suffered a variety of deprivations as a result. There will also have been considerable strain on the well parent from caring for the sick partner and from trying to fill both paternal and maternal roles. If they have not already recruited friends or relatives to help with the care of the children, the therapists should encourage the well partner to do so.

It is becoming increasingly common for people with schizophrenia and other severe psychiatric illnesses to meet in psychiatric facilities and form partnerships. Some will go on to have children, and we have already worked with several such families.

Clinical example
A daughter describes how she and her sister manage: both parents met in hospital.
Daughter. Mum's had problems. So has dad sometimes. We just have to manage. Some days are fine, and my sister visits when she can. I did leave home 18 months ago. But it didn't work out. Mum came round and phoned up all the time, so I moved back in.

The children of such partnerships have massive obstacles to overcome in order to achieve normal development, not the least of which is the dawning realisation that their parents are not like other children's parents. These children will have been designated as at risk from the beginning of their lives, with a consequent involvement of social services. However, there is still likely to be work for the therapists to undertake on the current understanding the children have of their parents' illnesses. Even where only a single parent, usually a mother, is ill, again social services will be intimately involved with the family and a decision will have been taken shortly after each child's birth over whether to keep mother and child together.

Sometimes a child will have been removed from a mother with schizophrenia and placed with another relative by social services. This may be a grandparent or sibling of the patient. A tense relationship can develop between the patient and relative over the care of the child, corresponding to other 'tug-of-love' situations. This is often made worse by the relative citing the patient's illness as a reason to criticise her mothering ability. Of course, there may be a basis for this, but if the relative is found to be critical of or hostile to the patient, that person will need to be worked with like any other high-EE relative.

Exposure of the child to symptoms

Some patients are able to keep their delusions and hallucinations to themselves except when acutely ill. Others find it hard to contain the experiences and are prone to talk to any family member about them, or even to people outside the family. Children exposed to a parent's delusions or hallucinations are likely to be very upset and frightened by them. They may not have been able to formulate them as symptoms of an illness. Therapists should allow children to express their feelings concerning the symptoms their parent has told them about, and should be given an understandable illness model to fit them into. It is not uncommon for children to develop a feeling of responsibility for the parent's illness, and for them to attribute it to their own bad behaviour. This needs to be thoroughly explored and appropriate reassurance and explanation provided.

As with adult relatives, children may find it difficult to view negative symptoms as part of an illness. Furthermore, they may be affected by having an inactive, emotionally unresponsive parent as a role model. The positive aspects of the ill parent should be emphasised and the children helped to relate to them. They may need another role model of the same sex as the ill parent to assist them with their own development.

Factors influencing the child's response to a parent with schizophrenia

The course of the parent's illness clearly has an important effect. With intermittent illnesses, the child can experience the parent as being relatively well between episodes and can learn to identify the behaviour that is part of the illness. However, if the illness is continuous, the child has a much more difficult task in distinguishing those aspects of the parent that are healthy from those that are sick. This is something that the therapists can provide assistance with.

The patient's degree of insight is also important, as it will determine the extent to which the pathological experiences are shared with the children.

The partner's attitude will influence the children's approach to the sick parent. If the partner is critical or hostile, the children may adopt the same attitude or may attempt to defend the sick parent. An overinvolved partner may collude with the patient's delusions or hallucinations, increasing the children's difficulty in establishing reality testing.

Another dimension is added to the problem if the children are incorporated into the parent's delusional system, for example by becoming the object of paranoid or sexual delusions. Under these circumstances, separation of the children from the sick parent should be seriously considered.

Specific problems

Parental conflict

This is relatively common in high-EE families, and there is always the risk that it will lead to violence. Children in the household are likely to be frightened by the threat or actuality of violence between their parents. Therapists will always take a firm line against the escalation of conflict, but this is even more important when there are young children present.

Parental absence

The inevitable absences of a sick parent due to hospital admissions are certain to have an effect on children. The healthy parent should be encouraged to take the children to visit the other parent in hospital, with suitable preparation about the nature of the ward. Sometimes children develop a fear that the sick parent will be taken away forever. Visits to the parent in hospital can be reassuring.

Unfortunately, suicide is common in schizophrenia, the lifetime rate being about 10%. If this tragedy occurs, the surviving parent may not be in a state of mind to deal with the children's grief and need to mourn. The therapists may need to attend to this or refer the children to an appropriate specialist.

Parental preoccupation

The needs of the sick adult may take up a lot of the healthy partner's emotional energy, which in turn may affect parenting ability and lead to emotional deprivation of the children. Furthermore, one of the children, usually the oldest, may take on a parenting role in relation to the other siblings. There may also be pressure on one or more of the children to act in a parental role towards the sick parent. Premature parenting is likely to interfere with the normal emotional development of a child. The therapists may be able to deal with this problem by changing the balance of care in the family, but sometimes a child may need referral to the appropriate psychiatric facility.

A related problem is the need children may perceive to protect their parent's reputation and authority against the teasing of other children at school. It will be helpful in this instance for the therapists to discuss with the family the origins of stigma and the reasons why people need to make fun of the mentally ill. It can be useful to request the child's head teacher or class teacher to initiate discussion in the school on this topic. The therapists should be prepared to offer some input into such a discussion.

Concern about inheritance or contagion

Older children may express a fear of catching mental illness or may be worried about inheritance. A frank discussion of the risks to children of a parent with schizophrenia (about 8%) should be offered by the therapists. This should be couched in terms that the children will understand. Some children may worry about passing the illness on to their own offspring. They can be reassured that the risk is no more than 2%, that is, twice the risk in the general population.

Summary

Children who have a parent with schizophrenia are likely to face a variety of problems to do with impaired parenting. This may result from the direct effect of the illness on the parent with schizophrenia or the indirect effect on the healthy parent. Children will have to cope with absences when the parent is in hospital and possibly with exposure to the symptoms of schizophrenia. The therapists need to provide them with an age-appropriate explanation of the illness. Family work can help children resolve their problems but they may require referral to a child guidance clinic.

CHAPTER 20

Carers who are siblings or children

Occasionally the main carer in a household is a sibling of the patient or an adult child. There are problems specific to these relationships which are not shared by parents or partners. In this chapter, in addition to these problems, we will also consider the emotional responses of siblings to a person with schizophrenia, even when they have no obvious caring role.

Siblings

Emotional responses

There are a number of emotional reactions that therapists need to be aware of in attempting to strengthen the sibling's caring role or to recruit the sibling to help the patient to become more independent. One of the commonest is shame and embarrassment: the sibling does not want friends to be aware of the patient's illness, for fear of being stigmatised or mocked. Fear of developing the illness can stem from a false belief about contamination or a correct knowledge of the pattern of inheritance. On the other hand, healthy siblings may suffer from 'survivor guilt', wondering why they escaped while their sibling is suffering. There can be a fear of having to take over the caring role when the parents die. Siblings may feel envious of the extra attention the patient gets from the parents and resentful of their own relative neglect. Related to this may be anger that the patient can get away with behaviour that they were punished for.

These negative emotions often lead siblings to distance themselves from the household, spending as much time away as possible, even when they still live with their parents. However, therapists should always consider healthy siblings as potential allies. They are often able to comment on the family's relationships in a relatively objective way and much more directly and forcefully than the therapists would risk. They act as good role models for the patient, particularly when they have managed to achieve an independent life. They are potentially able to introduce the patient to a group of people of their own generation, which is obviously more appropriate than the patient sharing social activities with the parents. For all these reasons, it is worth trying to engage siblings in family sessions, even when they are living apart. There is usually a fund of goodwill towards the patient that can be tapped, if the negative emotions can be aired and adequately dealt with. It is often valuable to hold sessions with the patient and siblings together, to which the parents are not invited. This strategy also emphasises respect for intergenerational boundaries.

Clinical example
A brother related, in front of the patient, that he used to hate him and wished he would die. This was because the patient would sit on the stairs with a kitchen knife, so that the brother was too frightened to go up to his bedroom. He said he spent as much time as possible out of the house with his friends and did not tell them about his brother. However, after some time he decided to share his problems with them. They were very sympathetic and now kept the patient company while the brother went out.

The caring role

Siblings are typically not as committed to the patient as are parents, who have cared for the patient since childhood, or partners, who have chosen their relationship. We have rarely encountered an overinvolved sibling, but siblings can be highly critical. In the normal course of their development, siblings would be expected to develop heterosexual relationships of their own outside the household. They may feel inhibited from doing this by the demands that the patient's care makes on them, or by their reluctance to acquire something that is out of the patient's reach. This can lead to resentment of the patient and a critical attitude.

Clinical example
A brother talks about having to look after his youngest sister.
Mr A.   We've always been together. I've always had to look after her. It's just been a
         duty, something that I've had to take on once our mother died. It's not as if I had
         a choice. I've just had to put up with how difficult she can be.

The therapists' aims are to reduce the responsibility siblings take for the patient and encourage them to attend to their own needs. In parallel with this, the therapists need to build up the patient's confidence in looking after him-/herself. Sometimes siblings find themselves thrust into the role of carer through the death of parents, as in the above example. They may feel guilty about their previous intention to be as uninvolved with the patient as possible and swing to the other extreme in trying to replace the parents. If they are married, their partner is likely to be resentful of the new focus of attention. The therapists' task is to make siblings feel that their efforts are valued but to moderate the amount they try to do for the patient, and to develop the patient's sense of autonomy. It may be difficult to persuade siblings to give up some of their responsibility for the patient if they have chosen this as their role in life, and particularly if they have some moral backing for it, for instance 'duty as a Christian'.

Children

When a parent suffers from schizophrenia, adult children are likely to show different attitudes and adopt varying roles. One at least will probably accept a caring role, though it depends a great deal on how able the other parent is to fulfil this function. If the other parent is physically or mentally ill, or absent for some reason, the whole burden is likely to fall on one of the children. The response can be to take over a parental role completely and to show overinvolved behaviour and attitudes. This is likely to entail poorly expressed feelings, particularly resentment at having to relinquish the role of a child in the family prematurely. The carer may also experience the loss of a parent as a source of advice and guidance, and may lack an adequate role model for parenting. Therapists should be prepared to help the carer with grieving for the 'lost' parent and resentment about the untimely role reversal.

These carers are likely to experience anxieties about ever being able to live their own life or to leave to set up a family of their own. The therapists need to address the usual issues of giving the carer permission to relinquish some responsibility for the sick parent and helping to relieve guilt. If there are other siblings around, the therapists should try to recruit them to share some of the responsibility, and thus give the caring child respite. If no other sibling is available, professional agencies should be brought in to give the carer some relief. As always, work should be directed towards helping patients become more able to look after themselves.

Summary

Siblings are likely to have complex negative feelings about the patient. However, there is usually a degree of goodwill that can be tapped to engage siblings in family work. They have the potential to be very useful allies in helping the patient towards independence. Siblings who are carers may have dedicated their life to looking after the patient, while adult children are likely to experience anxieties about being imprisoned in the caring role. In both instances, the therapeutic aim is to increase the patient's capacity for independence and to relieve the carer of some of the burden of responsibility.

CHAPTER 21

Employment

Helping patients to gain outside employment or return to education

The effect of schizophrenia can be very crippling, particularly for those patients with negative symptoms. Some patients may never have had the experience of employment for any length of time if the illness started during adolescence. In any case, starting a new job or returning to full-time education after a long absence can be stressful for anyone. It is a big step, with a significant risk of relapse if not handled carefully. In a relatives' group, suggestions can be made by other people regarding how to interest a patient in an occupation.

Clinical example

T.   What sort of jobs is Richard going for?
Mrs A. Does he fancy library work? It's easy sitting at a desk.
Mrs B. Is he interested in any adult education?
Mrs C. He has ideas one minute and the next morning he doesn't want to.
Mr B.   I go to a woodwork thing. It's very easy going. They don't do anything like that?
Mrs C. He keeps on joining evening classes.
Mr B.   No, I meant during the day.
T.   When did he last try? Why don't you suggest it to him?

The skills necessary to be in employment or education are complex. They include good time keeping, tolerance of some sort of routine, a large degree of independence while away from home, reasonable motivation to do well, the ability to pay attention to details, the ability to understand and incorporate advice or feedback from supervisors or teachers, and the ability to communicate and mix with fellow workers or pupils. Hence it should be attempted only if patients have been stable for several months and everyone in the family agrees to it, so that other family members can provide support and take part in problem solving. Furthermore, patients and family members should be able to recognise early signs of the illness and be able to deal with them. Some families may be impatient and want patients to go back to work or school and get on with life. Others might be hesitant, perhaps because of past experience that patients may not be able to bear the stress, and relapse, requiring the family to deal with the illness all over again. In either case, the family should be persuaded to adopt the graded behavioural approach discussed in Chapter 8.

Preparation of patients

Because of the complexity of skills required for employment or education, preparation should be over a period of time. It is worth being alert to the idea of 'making up for lost time'. Patients can enter a vicious circle of getting back to employment or full-time education prematurely and hence relapsing. It is a good idea to frame starting work or education as a trial, so that failures can be put into context.

A behavioural approach of small steps with increasing difficulty tailored to the individual is useful. To begin with, chores at home can be used as practice for concentration, independence, taking responsibility and tolerance of routine. As time goes by, the number of tasks and the length of time needed can be increased gradually. Homework practice can also involve patients getting up at a specified time to accomplish particular tasks. Attendance at day centres for industrial or educational programmes is good practice for time keeping, tolerance of routine, and sticking to jobs outside the home before patients finally face the world outside. Therapists should be prepared to provide support and be available during this difficult period.

An immediate issue when applying for jobs is whether to tell potential employers about past psychiatric history. There is no clear-cut answer to that problem. The advantage of telling the truth is that employers may be more supportive or sympathetic, particularly during a time of stress. However, the danger is that it will jeopardise the patient's chance of employment. Some employers may not consider employing someone with a significant past psychiatric illness at all. Hence some patients prefer to gloss over the issue. Whatever happens, it has to be a decision made by patients themselves. A discussion about the pros and cons with family members present will enable patients to make an informed decision.

As usual, families should be warned of the difficulties and complexity involved so that they can be prepared for setbacks. To begin with, a part-time job or returning to education part time may be less risky than a full-time occupation. Some patients, because of negative symptoms or a deterioration in skills, may have to look for a less ambitious job than they had previously. This may create problems for both patients and other family members, particularly if they come from a professional background. It may take a lot of discussion and exploration of feelings for them to come to terms with the fact that patients may not be as capable or skilled as they used to be. However, most families are able to accept it in the end, particularly if it is emphasised that patients have to make a start to re-establish their careers.

The development of social firms (cooperative enterprises run jointly by patients and staff) is a promising innovation. Social firms provide positions of responsibility which some patients can manage and appreciate, and bring patients into contact with the general public through the services offered by the firm.

For patients with severe disability, it may not be realistic to expect them to be able to get back to work. Even for those with less disability, whether they can return to paid employment depends on the economic climate. It can be virtually impossible to get a job during a deep recession. In these circumstances, unpaid work will have to be considered. Furthermore, therapists may have to help the families of patients with severe disability to define 'work' broadly. Just as running a home can be defined as full-time employment, a patient's contribution to the running of the home can be seen as 'work'. Sometimes, particularly in the marital home with the wife employed full time, the patient's contribution to running the home can be valued. Similarly, attendance at a day centre can be construed as work.

In a relatives' group it is possible to share the problem of helping a patient back into some structured activities, despite negative symptoms. Therapists' and other relatives' recognition and encouragement of the effort involved is important to help relatives maintain their input.

Clinical example
T1. Do you feel you've been quite successful in getting David up and to the hospital each day?
Mrs A.   Well it has been successful, but I don't know if it served any good purpose. He's not gone to the hospital and done anything.
T2. Well it is good for him.
T1. It gets him into a bit of a routine.
Mrs B.   [To Mrs A] You need to keep emphasising that.
T1. He's not just staying at home all day.

Summary

A behavioural approach to the performance of tasks at home by the patient gives the opportunity to exercise skills needed in a job. When applying for jobs, patients face the dilemma of how much to reveal of their psychiatric history. There is no clear-cut answer, but the therapists should discuss the pros and cons with the patient and the family. Families may need help in adjusting to the patient's impaired work skills and the reduced likelihood of finding open employment or returning to full-time studies. For patients with severe disability, families will have to be persuaded to accept alternatives such as helping out at home or attending a day centre.

CHAPTER 22

Cultural issues

All large cities in Britain contain peoples of ethnic minorities who have migrated more or less recently. Some will have found it relatively easy to assimilate into the majority White culture. Others strongly maintain their culture of origin and resist pressures to assimilate. Therapists need to be aware of the range of cultures they are likely to come into contact with in their work with families, and must cultivate sensitivity to those cultural issues that have a direct bearing on the work.

Language

This is the most obvious factor that may constitute an insuperable barrier to family work. If one of the key family members is able to speak English only poorly or not at all, the ideal solution is to find a therapist who can speak the family's language. Failing this, it is possible to use an interpreter who is not a member of the family. However, this has the disadvantages of slowing down communication and of inhibiting the family's responses, because of the presence of a stranger whom they might not trust. For example, they could worry that the interpreter might meet them later in a social setting, which is quite likely if the ethnic community is small. The alternative of using family members as interpreters is also problematic, since they may have reservations about representing the opinions of someone they disagree with. Hence the therapists could be given a censored version. Since both these solutions have disadvantages, the therapists need to weigh one against the other in making a decision.

Even when the therapists speak the same non-English language as the family, there can be difficulties in translating the concepts used in this work from English to the other language. Therapists should be aware of this difficulty and will need to check the family's understanding of particular concepts, by asking for feedback.

Ethnic matching of therapists with clients

Even if the family is fluent in English, it has been proposed by some that therapists should be chosen with a similar cultural background to that of the clients. In most services it is difficult to match therapists with recent immigrant groups because it takes some years for members of such groups to work their way onto and up the professional ladder. Even with well-established ethnic minorities, there is unlikely to be sufficient flexibility in the service to consider ethnic matching because of a general shortage of staff and in particular of those from the relevant ethnic group. The most practical solution is to ensure that all therapists are well versed in the cultural issues discussed in this chapter.

Family structure

The structure of the family in the majority White culture in Britain has changed dramatically over the past 100 years. Large extended families, which were common in the Victorian era, have shrunk to the nuclear family with two parents and two children. Even the nuclear family has been eroded, as currently 40% of marriages end in divorce and almost one in five families are headed by a single parent. Furthermore, 'blended' families, with children from different partners, are becoming more common. As a result of divorce or death of the partner, it is common to find one elderly parent, almost always the mother, looking after a middle-aged patient with schizophrenia by herself.

By contrast, many ethnic minority families retain a traditional structure, with large numbers of children and more distant relatives either sharing the household or otherwise being closely involved in their lives. Therapists must be prepared to hold family meetings with all adult members, including those in the extended family, since they may play an important role in supporting the patient.

In ethnic minorities, families tend not only to be larger but usually to be more hierarchical. The parents often expect respect and a sense of duty from their children. These values have all but vanished from White majority families, although some people can remember a time when sons addressed their fathers as 'Sir'. In some traditional families there are strict rules regulating communication. For instance, senior members must not converse with the most junior members except through an intermediary. Therapists should respect this structure, however different it is from their own experience.

The children in traditional families will often have been caught up in a conflict between the values of their family and those of the White majority culture, to which they will usually have been exposed at school. Therapists may be tempted to side with the children against the parents, but this should be resisted. They should do their best to give equal support to members of both generations, recognising that such conflicts are inevitable and that there may be no obvious solution.

One aspect of stronger parental authority that may impinge on family work is the arranged marriage. Often such marriages are arranged through other parents, and the prospective bride and groom may not meet until the wedding day. Sometimes traditional parents see this as the salvation for a son or daughter with schizophrenia and the mental illness may remain concealed throughout the marriage negotiations. The therapists need to raise the issue that marriage can be harmful or beneficial to the patient, depending on the nature of the relationship with the spouse. This cannot easily be predicted from parental knowledge of the two partners and is best determined by allowing them to spend some time together before the marriage is settled. However, therapists will often find themselves blocked by traditional values and customs.

The question of the appropriate age for children to become independent of their parents is also heavily influenced by culture. In traditional families, the children may be expected to stay with their parents throughout their life and to support them in their old age. Therapists must make allowance for this in setting goals for increased independence of the person with schizophrenia.

The structure of African-Caribbean families may be different from that of White majority families because of the nature of their immigration. It was quite common for the younger children to be left in the West Indies with grandparents and to join their parents in Britain some years later, when they had established themselves economically. Sometimes, by the time they joined the family, the parents had divorced and there was a step-parent and step-siblings. These disruptions in family relationships can cause emotional disturbances, to which the therapists should be sensitive.

Another feature of African-Caribbean families is that sometimes the adult men are not permanently resident in the household but come and go. This can be encountered with the husbands of women or the fathers of children affected with schizophrenia. Difficulties arise in engaging in family work men who are transient in this way. Nevertheless, persistent efforts should be made to do so.

Maintaining 'face'

In traditional cultures, particularly in Asia, a great deal of importance is attached to maintaining the family's respect in the eyes of neighbours, distant relatives and society in general. Mental illness is heavily stigmatised and the thought that its presence in a family member could become public knowledge is likely to raise anxieties about 'losing face'. It can also be seen as a blight on the marriage prospects of other children in the family. Hence the therapists have to approach education of the family tactfully and anticipate negative reactions to the diagnosis.

Beliefs about the causes and treatment of illness

Therapists should also be aware that the beliefs about mental illness held by traditional cultures often involve a causal role for spirits or fate. Acceptance of a Western biomedical model is consequently less likely than with families from the majority White culture. This should not deter therapists from working with the families on all other aspects of the programme, agreeing to disagree over the concept of schizophrenia.

It is likely to be more difficult to persuade relatives from traditional families to attend the relatives' group. Furthermore, they may be reluctant for the patient to attend facilities outside the home.

The advantages

Despite these difficulties it is important to remember that the outcome for schizophrenia in developing countries is considerably better than it is in the West, partly because of more tolerant attitudes of relatives. The extended family is a valuable resource for supporting patients with schizophrenia. Rather than feeling overwhelmed by the large families of ethnic minority patients, therapists should view them as a network of potential allies.

Summary

Cultural issues arise regularly in therapeutic work in cities. Language barriers require the use of an interpreter, but this is problematic in family work. Therapists have to take account of the variation in family structure and roles across cultures. Mental illness is more heavily stigmatised in families from developing countries. Although ethnic matching of clients and therapists may be ideal, it is often impractical. Therefore therapists need to develop sensitivity to cultural issues.

CHAPTER 23

Special problems complicating family work

Alcohol and substance misuse

The most common concerns with regard to substance misuse among families of patients with schizophrenia are problems relating to alcohol, cigarettes, soft drugs such as marijuana, street drugs such as crack and ecstacy, and excessive caffeine intake.

Clinical example
In this family alcohol and drug misuse were a problem.

T.   Do you think you are less well now than you have been Leslie, if you couldn't sleep all night?
P.   Well the Sudafed makes me, keeps me awake unless I've had a drink and taken some chlorpromazine.
T.   You seem shaky today as well.
M.   Then why do you take it? Is it meant to do you any good?
P.   There's a drug in it which is speed. It gives me my anxiety totally away from my self-conscious so I don't call on my subconscious.

Drugs and substance misuse are often an emotional issue. The evidence that certain ethnic groups are more likely to use soft drugs is equivocal. However, it is a common misconception among some relatives that the patient's illness started because he/she mixed in bad company and used drugs, and that the illness is entirely due to drug misuse. While it is true that soft drugs or other recreational drugs have the unfortunate effect of enhancing vulnerability to the onset of the illness or relapses, drugs on their own do not cause the schizophrenia. This should be made clear to patients and their families, so that patients do not get blamed for causing their illness. However, the danger of using recreational drugs should be made clear to patients. We find it useful to have routine educational sessions about the danger of drug use while patients are still in hospital, and then to reiterate the harmful effects during family sessions if the use of recreational drugs is a problem. Patients should be advised clearly against any drug or substance misuse.

Dual-diagnosis disorders (the combination of psychosis and substance misuse) require close collaboration between the service providers for psychosis and those for substance misuse. Some community staff have now been trained in the management of dual-diagnosis disorders, which are becoming more common with the increasing availability of street drugs.

Alcohol is a common problem. People with schizophrenia like visiting pubs, where they can blend into an environment that provides some sort of social stimulation, without it being too demanding for them. Furthermore, visiting pubs is part of the culture for certain sections of the population in Britain. Patients may not feel one of the crowd, going to pubs with friends, if they abstain completely from alcohol. Unfortunately, alcohol does potentiate the sedative effects of tranquillisers. Patients should be warned about this as part of the educational process. A few patients become violent when demanding money for drinks or when drunk.

Complete abstinence may not be possible or necessary. Family members often worry about this and object to, or even try to take control of, the situation. This is unlikely to be successful without the patient's cooperation. As with any problems families have, patients' and relatives' concerns and points of view should be voiced in meetings. Patients and families should be helped to see the potential problems relating to alcohol intake and yet not lose sight of the opportunities to socialise with limited alcohol intake. Patients then should be helped to experiment with how much alcohol they can take without getting intoxicated. We often advise patients to order half pints rather than full pints of beer when going out in a crowd. Low-alcohol beer is a good alternative.

Clinical example
In this session the double problem of drug taking and drinking had been worked on.
T.   Last time we met we talked about how to organise the weekend. We compromised on Leslie going to stay with you on Friday and Sunday. I was just wondering how it's been?
M.   The last weekend sort of took care of itself because Leslie didn't come up till Saturday. He was very good; he didn't drink either night.
T.   Wonderful.
M.   I think he was a lot better for it.
T.   What did you say to Leslie when he didn't drink?
M.   I think I was just very pleased that he didn't get drunk. We set that arrangement and he stuck by it and I shall say it in the future, no coming home if he drinks, because it's not good for him and not good for me.
T.   How did you find the weekend Leslie?
P.   All right.
The therapists are also making sure that both sides join in, note the progress and reinforce positive changes.

Cigarette smoking is another common concern, owing to hazards to physical health. Often the complaint is not the smoking as such but the danger of setting the house on fire when patients are smoking in bed, or untidiness associated with smoking. Patients often say they smoke because of boredom. The problem of physical dependence, the usual scenario of fellow patients smoking heavily and cigarettes being a central focus for social interaction among patients make giving up smoking difficult. Often the solution is to help families to set limits with regard to specific problem behaviour relating to smoking. For example, the practice of smoking in bed should be discouraged, particularly if the patient is taking large doses of tranquillisers. Limits should also be set with regard to the use and emptying of ashtrays if that is a problem.

Lastly, some patients drink an enormous amount of tea or coffee. This can lead to shakiness, nervousness, excitement, restlessness and sleep problems. It should be explained to patients that sometimes it is difficult to separate the effects of too much caffeine intake from anxiety or the schizophrenic process itself. The amount of caffeine intake should, therefore, be moderated.

Child physical and sexual abuse

This does not occur more frequently in families where one member suffers from schizophrenia, as far as we know, but during family work it is likely that an occasional family will have this as an additional problem. The important issue here, as with alcohol and substance misuse, is to separate the family problems caused by the illness from those caused by the abuse. If the abuse is in the past, this will be one of the main tasks of the family work.

If the abuse is current or not previously discovered, then other agencies should be called in, in the same way that therapists would with any family. Child abuse is a serious offence; evidence that it is occurring would have to be taken further and the children must be protected as far as possible. If this happens, then the family are bound to feel ambivalent about the therapists and it may not be possible to continue working with them. Even if work continues, the impact of calling in outside agencies will have to be discussed with the family.

Any 'secret', and sexual abuse is one of the most likely, causes a conflict of interest for therapists. If therapists are told a 'secret' that others in the family may not share, then it makes family work more difficult. We have often found that the 'secret' is known but that family members are not able to talk to each other about it. Apart from sexual abuse (when therapists have to act on the knowledge, despite issues of confidentiality and trust), the aim with most 'secrets' is to enable the confiding family member to discuss it more openly in a family meeting. If therapists can give support for this, often all family members will feel relief at the subject finally being aired.

In our experience, when child abuse has been a problem, the damage done to the marital and child relationships complicates the problems of schizophrenia and is particularly difficult to repair.

Suicide

In a condition such as schizophrenia the risk of suicide, both threatened and successful, is high, and most patients and families will have some experience of this. The lifetime risk among patients is 10%. Some families react by becoming excessively cautious and overprotective. Others will not believe that the patient is serious and may underestimate the risks. If a relationship is particularly poor, or the family particularly burdened, relatives may even wish that the patient were dead – we have heard this said both in a relatives' group and in front of the patient during a family meeting.

If this happens, therapists have to interrupt the meeting and immediately comment on and reframe the remarks. We have found that even brutal-sounding statements like these can be looked at positively. They are also quite likely to have been said before, and are probably less shocking to other family members than to therapists. In this particular example, in the family meeting it was possible for therapists to comment on the fact that a relative felt like this because of concern that the patient's quality of life was so poor that she would be better off dead. The patient was then able to reassure the relative about it and appreciate the concern. In a relatives' group, several relatives admitted wishing the patient dead, and similar reasons were elicited – that is, fears that patients' lives now were almost unbearable. Once voiced, it was possible for relatives to discuss with and reassure each other that there were still positive aspects about the patients they lived with.

It is helpful to establish, with the family and the patient, the reality of suicidal feelings and possible actions. Patients may well have warning signs of these feelings – either as part of a relapse, or as part of new feelings of depression. Often, as the positive symptoms of schizophrenia decrease and patients return to some appreciation of reality, they may also be faced with severe feelings of loss and hopelessness – that they will never recover fully and that life will always be more difficult from now on. If a patient can share such feelings and possible warning signs, or relatives are familiar with them, then the action that can and should be taken can be rehearsed with the family. If it is possible to do this before a crisis arises, it will help to defuse the anxiety of a real crisis and enable relatively quick action to be taken. Depending on the local services, it may be helpful to suggest a telephone call to the general practitioner, the mental health team or the emergency services if the family or the patient are very concerned.

If patients become depressed or hopeless, they may need individual help. It may be necessary to discuss the fact of lowered expectations and help them to come to terms with it. A useful technique is 'collapsing time' (mentioned in Chapter 13), to discuss how they can make progress in a very long time span such as one or two years – it may be possible to look back over previous years to find evidence of this. For example, "Do you remember five years ago, when you were always in hospital?"

A successful suicide will be an especially devastating event for the therapists if they are working with the family at the time. Relatives will feel considerable anger and, of course, be extremely upset. Often the relatives will feel somebody is to blame. Normally there will be a hospital inquiry, an inquest and possibly court proceedings. Not all suicides are preventable and therapists need to remember this. Normally staff and relatives will have tried to prevent the death and this will have been documented. On the other hand, all involved will feel guilty and upset that prevention was not possible for whatever reason. Therapists are likely to be distressed and shaken themselves. They may also feel anger and resentment at the patient for causing such distress.

These situations are difficult to deal with. It helps if therapists are as open and understanding as possible with relatives, even if the family are angry. It can defuse things if therapists can say that they, too, are shocked and sad. Some families require contact and want to meet to discuss what happened; others will cut off and not want to have to deal with psychiatric staff anymore. The family's wishes have to be respected. We have found that if no other contact is wanted, a short letter of sympathy can still be helpful.

Similar principles apply if the death is not suicide but due to some other cause. Therapists will be upset and the family is unlikely to want to continue contact. Again, a short letter of sympathy can be helpful and may be easier to manage than a telephone call.

The family's permission must be sought if staff wish to attend the funeral, which is usually welcomed. The offer of continuing sessions or attendance at a relatives' group should be made, but it may not be taken up. In a relatives' group, a death needs to be discussed openly with group members, and will obviously raise fears of vulnerability and of what may happen in the future for other members.

Physical disabilities

It is quite common to find that patients (or relatives) have physical disabilities that complicate the problems of schizophrenia. Sometimes physical problems predate the illness, so that the patient has always had to have special care or help, and this can mark the start of an overinvolved relationship with a parent. Sometimes physical difficulties start at the same time as schizophrenia. For some patients, physical problems arise because of damage done during suicide attempts. Others have physical problems that arise later.

The aim here is to separate out the physical from the mental problems. Both the patient and their family may not understand the difference and the family may over- or underprotect the patient as a result. Once in the 'invalid' role, patients may not wish to be independent and may lose confidence in their abilities. One patient who needed lengthy physical treatment lost all community skills because of being 'looked after' in a general hospital and had to be encouraged over many months to go out of the house again.

Often, physical treatments, for example for diabetes, continue alongside treatment for mental health. Being involved with two teams can lead to confusion and therapists should be able to liaise with the other team and act as advocates for the patient and relatives if necessary. Patients with negative symptoms can have serious motivational problems in taking long-term treatment for physical problems and in attending clinics. This can be discussed in the family meetings and then dealt with as other problems would be.

More than one person in the family with schizophrenia

This is not common, but we have come across and worked with such families. Most typically, both partners in a marriage meet in hospital, and although it is likely that one is better, and is actually the carer, therapists may find that there is not a 'well' relative to deal with in family sessions. We have also met families where a parent and a child have schizophrenia, and other families where more than one child is ill.

Usually in these situations, only one person is the 'patient' for the therapists, and other family members will be seen by other teams. Sometimes, however, it will be sensible for both relatives to be 'patients'. This can lead both to a conflict of interest for therapists and to the patients feeling that only one of them (the more needy one) is getting help. Therapists need to be aware of this and to make sure that both parties feel well attended to.

Because schizophrenia is a diverse condition, two sufferers in the same family may have very different patterns from each other. This leads to confusion for both patients and relatives, with comments such as "I've managed to cope with my voices; why can't you?" The different severities of schizophrenia and even the possibility of different treatment regimes need to be explained by therapists, and help given according to what the problems are at the time. Occasionally the better 'patient' can be used as an ally to help the worse one, but often they are rather resentful of the attention given, and a positive response cannot be relied upon. Well members of the family, if they are available (and it may be necessary to involve the whole network), are particularly important to include and mobilise in family meetings in order to encourage healthy behaviour. Sometimes, a previously undiagnosed family member will volunteer psychotic symptoms and his/her own coping responses. It can be reassuring for patients to know that they are not unique in having strange experiences. However, although personally successful, the suggested solutions are often idiosyncratic and may not be helpful or acceptable to the patient. Therapists should take such suggestions seriously and allow them to be discussed, but establish that patients have to make their own decisions and may not share identical problems with other family members.

Working with several other agencies

As has been mentioned, some families are involved with more than one team. Sometimes this is because there are multiple problems in the family, as discussed under Physical disabilities, above; sometimes families attract multi-agency input because they are demanding of, or are dissatisfied with, services.

Therapists in this situation should be aware that the opportunities for misinformation, divisions arising between professionals and an uncoordinated approach multiply with the number of agencies. It is worth remembering that if a family complains of the 'other' team to therapists, they may be equally dissatisfied with family meetings. It is sensible to check directly with the other agency what their viewpoint is, or what their aims are with the family, rather than just accepting the family view.

If possible, one agency should provide the major input to a family and other agencies should channel through and liaise with them. If other therapists are already doing some family work, it would not be sensible to start sessions with the family as well, and some discussion should take place as to which therapists are going to continue and who should withdraw. The potential for sabotage and confusion makes it too difficult to offer family work in 'competition' with another agency. As soon as possible, a meeting should be called of all professionals involved with the family, with the aim of rationalising the input and ensuring that there is no overlap or cross-purposes.

Another possibility is that therapists discover the involvement of another agency only after several sessions – the family omit to mention it at first. Again, therapists need to talk to the other workers directly and negotiate with them.

Families who reject therapists

It does happen that despite families being well engaged with meetings and attending sometimes for months, therapists are told not to come again. This will feel rejecting for the therapists, who may also be quite shocked and angry with the family for making such a sudden decision. They have to accept what the family proposes, but should try to find out what the problem is. If it is something specific, it may be possible for the therapists to change their approach or deal with the problem and all may be well. However, some families become adamant on being questioned and the situation may not improve. If this is the case, therapists should try to negotiate a 'final session' in order to say goodbye and to do some work on leaving. Even if both sides are quite upset and angry, a final session, arranged for a few weeks' time, will allow for a cooling-off period. This in itself may encourage a different perspective by the next visit. If the family is still adamant, however, therapists should aim to be constructive in the 'goodbye' session. Progress should be reviewed and coping strategies rehearsed for any emergencies. Therapists should leave open the possibility that they can be contacted (e.g. by leaving a telephone number), even if this is rejected by the family at the time. It is important for therapists not to show that they are overly perturbed by the family's rejection of them. They should say that they would like to see the family again if they change their mind, and should wish them well for the future. Often this 'lifeline' will in fact be used. Another strategy is for therapists themselves to telephone 'for a chat' in a few weeks' time. This establishes that the therapists are still willing to be involved and are still concerned, and it can allow a reappraisal of any current problems.

Being rejected by the family will not feel comfortable for the therapists and they should talk it over together. When it does happen, the reason is likely to be that the family find change too difficult at that time and so end the sessions to protect themselves.

Summary

It is not uncommon to find that families are not coping just with schizophrenia but are also facing a range of other problems that may cause as much or even more concern. These include alcohol or substance misuse, child abuse, suicide attempts, physical disabilities and more than one family member affected by mental illness. Where there are multiple problems, the therapists need to help the family sort out the issues involved and deal with them adequately. Families sometimes reject the help offered. When this happens it is important for the therapists to offer them the possibility of future contact.

CHAPTER 24

Running a relatives' group. I

Relatives groups can be very hard work and therapists are likely to need considerable persistence to overcome problems such as poor attendance. The pros and cons of running a group should be carefully considered.

Advantages of relatives' groups

(a) Relatives' groups are cost-effective. Two therapists can work with 10 to 12 relatives in one group.
(b) They provide a good forum to express, process and normalise feelings, especially negative ones that would perhaps upset patients if they were exposed to them.
(c) The presence of other relatives creates the social pressure of a peer group who understand the problems. Furthermore, relatives (compared with professionals) can be very frank and forceful with each other without causing offence.
(d) A wider variety of solutions to difficult problems are likely to be proposed by a group than by a family, especially if there is only a single relative.
(e) Groups can expand relatives' social networks, which are often reduced by living with schizophrenia. They help to relieve the isolation and feelings of guilt and stigma.

Disadvantages of relatives' groups

(a) A group does not allow therapists to observe interaction between patients and relatives, which can deepen the therapists' understanding of the problems.
(b) Therapists get to hear only one viewpoint – the relatives'.
(c) A group cannot deal with worries that relatives feel are too private or intimate to be aired, such as marital or sexual problems.
(d) 'Newer' relatives may be upset by meeting relatives with very long-term problems.

(e) Some relatives will not attend a group, so that by itself a group will fail to offer a service to all families. In particular, those difficult to engage, people who are infirm or have a disability, the elderly and relatives who cannot manage the time of the meeting will be neglected. Our research has shown that patients have a poor outcome in families who are offered the group but fail to attend (Leff et al, 1989). These families should be offered individual family sessions.

General issues

One of the main features distinguishing relatives' groups from the family work described previously is that patients are not involved. This arrangement allows relatives to feel unconstrained enough to discuss a range of emotional aspects with other people in the group. Relatives are relieved by this; however, there is now some evidence that single-family interventions are more effective for patients than multi-family groups.

A relatives' group also immediately creates a problem in that patients may feel excluded, and some will be suspicious and upset at the prospect of relatives attending a separate meeting. We have found that saying the following to patients will reassure all but the most paranoid:

(a) that relatives themselves need help;

(b) that it is useful to meet with others who understand the problem;

(c) that we are not discussing the patients so much as trying to ensure that relatives cope better.

Clinical example

In one relatives' group, members discuss how to cope with a patient's worries about what is said in a meeting.

T.   What do you say to your husband?

Mrs Y.   Everything. Absolutely.

Mr X.   [To Mrs Y] Do you think I ought to go home and tell my wife?

Mrs Y.   She's obviously feeling a bit left out, even though she's the cause of it, perhaps even jealous that you belong to a group. One way round it is to let her know you've been helped a lot by hearing other people's experiences. You could say, "A lot of them are like you dear, but it's just nice to hear other people talking about someone ill with them." You could describe to her what some of us are like.

Mr X.   I find being cross-examined about what happened here embarrassing.

Mrs Y.   You needn't say anything about what you said. She might feel more included if you tell her about us. Let's say you go home and I'm you. And you say "There's a new girl there today, because her husband's been admitted really psychotic", maybe she might feel …

Mrs Z.   Better about it, not extraordinary.

Another feature of relatives' groups is that therapists have to work particularly hard to persuade people to attend. Unlike meetings in the home, relatives' groups must be held at a central location and this means that everybody has to travel. Since many relatives are elderly, have a disability, are unwell or are in employment, there is always a problem of motivation and often a problem over timing – for example, an evening group will suit those in work but not those who are elderly or infirm and dislike going out at night. It is also difficult to engage people in a new venture that requires meeting unknown people to discuss issues that were previously felt to be private and perhaps stigmatised. We have found that between a quarter and a half of potential relatives will not attend a group even when offered lifts and after letters reminding them of each meeting. Although, as mentioned above, it is cost-effective, it will always be the case that not all families will attend. These families will need sessions at home, since therapists on a doorstep are hard to refuse, whereas going out on a winter evening is easily avoided.

In order to maximise engagement we recommend that, if possible, therapists should meet relatives before a group is set up. Often this can be done by giving relatives the education package at home. It is less daunting to attend a group if relatives at least know the therapist.

Finally, when asked, relatives often say they would like 'talks' – that is, information and education provided as a set part of the meeting. When we have tried this, 'medication' was the most popular topic by far and the local pharmacy department provided very good input here. However, these more educational meetings may make it more difficult to work on problem solving and deal with emotional issues; we do not have evidence that this format, although appealing, actually improves outcomes.

Venue

Ideally the venue should be convenient, accessible, already known to the relatives and welcoming. There may be an argument for taking the group away from a mental health setting and organising it in a local community centre; however, this is likely to work only if relatives are already used to attending there for some other reason. Some relatives have suggested holding the group in a building close to shops and other facilities such as a pub. The room used should be comfortable, large enough to manage up to, say, 15 people, but not so huge as to be intimidating. We have always provided refreshments at meetings, so access to a kitchen and tea-making facilities is essential. The latter emphasises the social as well as the emotional needs of carers and helps members to feel relaxed. As increasing the social network is likely to be an aim of a relatives' group, this aspect is more important than it may seem initially.

Timing

As mentioned earlier, timing is not likely to suit everyone and should be negotiated if at all possible. We have usually held groups in the afternoon or early evenings; the former suits the elderly and retired, the latter those in work. The groups normally last for an hour and a half and are typically run once a fortnight, particularly if most families are at the beginning of the illness. For families of very long-term patients, we have found that once a month is a better frequency as new issues are less likely to arise.

Selection

Our main criterion for inclusion in these groups is having a relative with schizophrenia. If different diagnoses are included, patients' problems are not similar enough and it is difficult for the group members to develop themes and to feel that others understand their difficulties. The more similar members are, the easier it will be to develop common strategies that they will accept from each other. Most relatives will be parents, some will be partners and others will be siblings or children. If there are at least two of each sort, it will help the group to feel that they share experiences; if this is not possible, the therapists will have to work harder to make sure that the only partner or only father does not feel marginalised.

The only other aspect that we ensure is that all relatives have received the education (see Chapter 5) before the group starts. This gives the members a common base and it means that one of the therapists is likely to have met them already. Giving the education first also means that therapists have already provided relatives with something they wanted – information – and this is likely to increase their motivation to attend.

Size

If there are more than 12 people in the group, it will be difficult to attend to and give support for everyone's needs. Too few people will mean that the group is hardly viable: therapists will be effectively holding individual sessions. A group of up to, say, 15, of whom 7 to 10 will regularly attend, seems to be about the right size.

Open or closed groups?

We have always run an open group, mainly because of the difficulties of recruiting. Thus, relatives can start attending a group, continue it, preferably for about nine months, and then leave; they will then be replaced by other members. This has the advantage of new members introducing variety. It also allows relatives of people at different stages of illness to join a group and see for themselves that even very difficult problems can be coped with and survived. However, the relatives of first-onset patients can find listening to long-term problems discouraging and they will need extra support in the group, and sometimes outside it, to deal with this. There is an argument for seeing all relatives of first-onset patients in a separate group, but it is unusual to find enough people at the same time to make this practical.

Aims of a relatives' group

These are:
(a) to help lower criticism and overinvolvement in relatives;
(b) to help relatives share experiences and process the emotional upset that they have had;
(c) to allow relatives to pool solutions to problems and help each other to try out new ways of coping with common difficulties;
(d) to increase relatives' social networks, to combat feelings of isolation and stigma.

These aims are achieved by encouraging relatives to talk to each other about their experiences, to share and thus normalise the emotional impact, and to allow relatives to solve common problems and try out new ways of coping that can be reinforced by the social approval of group members.

Clinical example
This discussion is about the possibility of a relapse.
T.   You're hoping it's going to be alright in the future, Mr A, because, as you say, last time it was a "nightmare" for you.
Mr A.   Oh if it happens again I'm off, I'm going, I'll ring up Dr T and say "I'm bailing out".
Mrs B.   I can understand that, because we went through hell.

Therapists' role

Although this is a group, the therapists do not rely on traditional or psychodynamic 'group processes'. The therapists' role is to facilitate the group members' interaction in order to allow them to achieve the above aims. Thus, many of the same tactics used with families are also required in the group. Relatives must 'take turns', listen to each other and not all talk at once. The atmosphere of the group must be friendly and positive, while also allowing serious issues to be tackled and problems solved. Relatives' groups are particularly good at dealing with the emotional processing that families may not have managed previously. Group members must be able to trust each other and the therapists enough to raise these issues. Upsetting emotions must be allowed to be expressed, normalised and used positively. The group must therefore be safe enough to enable this. Therapists must also take control and be directive enough to help members stick with one subject and manage to talk about an issue so that there is some productive conclusion, otherwise the members can avoid discussion of solutions and the time spent together will not help families to change their behaviour.

Summary

A relatives' group can look cost-effective but may not always be feasible. If it is established, therapists must work very hard to engage members and maintain attendance. A relatives' group requires similar skills to those discussed in the family sessions; the aims and methods are parallel. Therapists are primarily facilitators. Relatives need help to engage in the group, and patients may be suspicious of its purpose. The venue should be convenient and kitchen facilities should be available.

CHAPTER 25

Running a relatives' group. II

The first group meeting

It is important for the first meeting to help everyone to relax and to begin to get to know each other. Everyone should be welcomed and the therapists should introduce themselves as relatives arrive. In our experience, a good way to start the meeting is to ask all relatives to give a short version of their 'story', that is, their name, the patient's name and an account of what has happened to them since the illness began. Asking relatives to do this for themselves allows them to keep control of the story and to reveal only what they feel comfortable with. Even so, some may need encouragement to talk at all and the therapists should provide this. Relatives should be asked to talk in turn and therapists should ensure that they are listened to and not interrupted. This emphasises that turn taking and listening are important in the group, in the same way as they are in the family sessions. If one relative or one couple tells a very involved story and begins to dominate the meeting, the therapists should interrupt politely and say that the meeting will return to their problems later on or in a subsequent meeting; it is important that therapists establish from the start that everyone in the room should be given the chance to contribute.

As relatives begin to talk about their experiences, the group will begin to discover the similarities between them. Therapists should also emphasise these as they occur – "You just mentioned that, didn't you, Mrs X?" or "You felt like that too". This not only begins the process of 'communality' that is an important feature of these relatives' groups, but also makes the point that therapists have been listening and are able to draw out the themes.

The main aim of the first meeting is to establish how much all the participants have in common, despite differences in background or relationship. Relatives with some uncommon feature must be reassured by the therapists that their problem is not particularly unusual even if no one else in the group mentions it, otherwise they will feel isolated and it will be harder for them to attend next time. Therapists should ensure that everyone has a chance to participate and that each person's contribution is valued.

After the 'stories' have been heard, the focus should be on some experience that several relatives have had. This allows a discussion to develop and therapists should ask for everyone's view. It is important that therapists keep control during this sort of discussion, as it cannot be assumed that relatives will all have the same level of social and participatory skills. It will often be necessary to reinforce listening to each other, to emphasise that relatives must not interrupt too often and to make sure that only one person talks at a time. The last can be introduced as a 'rule' of the group, otherwise it is easy for relatives to try to have parallel conversations, either with each other or with each therapist, and the group will become chaotic.

We have found that having a break for tea and biscuits in the middle of the meeting works well. It allows relatives to enjoy the social side of a group, it helps people to relax and it emphasises that the group shares some of the characteristics of other meetings that they may have attended. Once the tea is served, however, we carry on with the meeting.

Subsequent meetings

After the first meeting, it is important that the therapists continue to have clear aims for the meetings and impose some structure on them, otherwise the group will soon feel repetitious and pointless. We would usually begin each subsequent meeting with an open enquiry to each relative as to how things had been since the last time. This allows any urgent or unexpected issues to be raised and looked at by the group. Any new group members should be introduced in the same way as in the first meeting – all group members can be asked for their 'story'. The new member is included in this exercise, although not necessarily asked to begin it, and this helps not only to introduce everybody but also allows the new person to join the group.

During each meeting the therapist should be alert to any theme or common problem that is being mentioned. Part of the point of the group is to allow members to focus on common issues that they probably previously thought were quite individual. This gives members not only a chance to 'normalise' their difficulties, but also, and even more important, to use the group to find new ways of coping. Thus, once a problem has been identified, the therapists' role is to enable members to discuss it in some depth, to stay with it and not stray off the point, and, finally, to come to some 'low-EE' consensus as to a possible solution. This can be extremely difficult to achieve if all group members have high-EE ratings, and this is one of the reasons we suggest having two therapists. Another strategy is to try to ensure that at least some low-EE relatives attend the group. They will be harder to engage, as their needs will be different, but if they do join the group, therapists can use their experiences of coping with problems as a realistic but alternative model. Low-EE relatives can be an asset in groups because they have had to cope with the same difficulties but have often found a more effective coping strategy.

Clinical example

Mrs A was very angry with her husband's demanding and irritable behaviour.

Mrs A.   It's part of this illness. They've got us there and there's nothing we can do about it. It sounds half the time that we let them have their own way; we do, but it's just to live in the same house with them. That's what it boils down to: we've got to live with these people and it doesn't matter how bitter and hurt you're feeling, we've got to tolerate their way of carrying on. Haven't you found that?

Mrs B.   Up to a point.

Mrs A.   Half the time you can say "What's your bloody game? Why did you do this?"

Mrs B.   I think acceptance is the great thing. What they say to you – you know damn well they're trying to irritate you or doing something like that.

Mrs A.   This is it.

Mrs B.   And you just have to let it ride.

Mrs A.   It's what you do eight out of ten times. It just seems so bloody unfair.

Mrs B.   You've got to do that, otherwise you'll always be at loggerheads. You have to let it ride, really, if you can possibly do it.

T.   What do you think Mr C?

Mr C.   I normally go out.

Mr B.   Don't give any backchat?

Mr C.   I have done, but over the years I've learnt that it doesn't avail anything at all, only upset myself. I just tolerate it now. If I talk to friends I can say what I like, because I know the person, but sometimes with my wife I have to think what I'm saying because she is hypersensitive and can take things to heart.

Mrs B.   That's right.

Mr C.   Thing's that wouldn't upset anyone else.

Themes

In early meetings of the group, while people are getting to know each other, most of the themes raised are likely to be practical. Relatives often ask a lot of questions, both of the therapist and of each other, that are related to the education session. Issues raised include medication (this is particularly likely), the causes of schizophrenia, employment, problems with benefits and practical problems caused by the patient. We recommend answering any questions as they arise and also at times throwing questions open to the whole group to elicit their answers. In most groups therapists will find that at least one relative will have had experience of the problem and will be likely to have a useful opinion. Part of the value of a relatives' group is that it is easier to listen to the opinions and advice of someone who has had the same experience, and it is also deeply reassuring to hear that someone else has coped with or learnt to live with very difficult and even intractable problems.

Later on, as more trust develops between group members, more difficult emotional issues will be raised. Groups provide a setting to deal with these: there are no patients present, so relatives feel they need not be constrained, and even negative emotions will have been felt by other group members. Typical issues will include the stigma of mental illness, feelings of isolation, grief, loss and bereavement. Relatives will often feel angry and may want to reject the patient or the caring role. The power of the patient to make relatives feel guilty, helpless or frightened may be raised.

Other emotional themes are the vulnerability of patients and relatives' fear of the future – "Who will look after the patient when I am gone?" There will usually also be discussion of services – often regarding how they have failed relatives, both in the past and currently. If this includes the therapists' own service, they should deal with the criticism calmly. It may be necessary to offer to act as an advocate to improve services. Something as simple as a telephone call by a therapist to a key worker or a consultant may make an appreciable difference to the way a family is dealt with.

Problem solving

As in the family sessions, if a problem is raised, attempts should be made during the group to solve it. If several problems are mentioned at the beginning of the meeting, then the therapists should attempt to prioritise them with the group members. Less urgent issues can always be deferred to a future meeting. Once a problem has been identified, possible solutions should be canvassed and discussed. Even reticent members should be asked for their views and encouraged to participate. The problem should be specified and broken into small, achievable bits, and the mechanics of any solutions should be discussed with the group in detail. If possible, a task should be agreed on and homework set, to be reported on next time. Any progress that is achieved can then be powerfully reinforced by the whole group at the next meeting.

Clinical example
A patient's needs for reassurance had been discussed earlier and the relatives' new response is reinforced by the group.
Mrs A.   Eve makes excuses to go to bed. She won't go up unless someone is there. I can't explain it.
T1.   What do you do now to reassure her?
Mr A.   Usually I say I'm going; I don't force her to go to bed now. I say we're going to bed.
T1.   So you leave her downstairs?
T2.   Quite right.
Mrs A.   I did once or twice creep down, but now she switches it all off herself.
Mrs B.   That's good.

Sometimes, relatives get into a 'catch-22' of being unable to try a new solution: "The problem is too difficult to have a solution. I have tried everything. Any new solution could not work (because it would mean that I am a failure), therefore there is no solution." Throughout the whole of the meeting they may argue this. Therapists should recognise this as a relative trying to avoid the uncertainty of change, and be reassuring. We have often found that relatives who do this will in fact manage a change between sessions and be able to report back about it with enthusiasm next time.

Emotional processing

When relatives do begin to express emotional issues, particularly the negative ones, it is important that therapists are able to cope. By being aired, the emotions are shared with the rest of the group, and this allows them to be normalised and put into context. Even extreme emotions will have been experienced by other group members, and others in the group will also be likely to have come to terms with them, or at least to have started the process. Therapists should use the group's experience in a positive way to show how even very upsetting and difficult feelings can lead to new ways of coping with and understanding problems. Therapists should also not be visibly shocked, even by very negative emotions, for instance wishing that a suicide attempt had been successful; by allowing such emotions to be expressed in the safety of the group setting, they are helping to defuse them and to reduce the likelihood of their being said to the patient. The burden of care can be shared in a group.

Clinical example
Mrs A.   I get very tired. I feel like walking out of the house and not coming back.
T1.   Why can't you do that – go for a walk but come back later?
Mrs A.   Because I can't. Because of the roads. I've got that problem as well.
Mrs B.   Have a long bath.
T1.   Haven't you got a neighbour you could go to?
T2.   It sounds as though you shut yourself away somewhere else.
Mrs A.   I just get depressed.
Mrs C.   I hide it from my daughter. I don't let her see I'm upset.
Mrs D.   You couldn't hide it from Diane.
T2.   If it makes you cry like that, perhaps you ought to let her know later on, that is, when you feel calmer; have a talk about how difficult it is.

Maintaining attendance

If group attendance falls, relatives who do turn up will begin to feel dispirited and the group will become non-viable. Therapists can maintain attendance by being consistent themselves, by being positive and encouraging to those who do attend, by reminding each relative by letter of the date of each meeting and, if necessary, by offering lifts to those relatives who are elderly or infirm.

Ending a group

Not all groups have an end. Some members may want to continue without a facilitator; sometimes therapists are able and willing to continue to run it. We have usually run a group for about two years. If it is going to end, it is important to give relatives plenty of warning and to discuss with them what support they would like in the future. Sometimes relatives have become friendly enough with each other to feel that they will not need extra help – we have had relatives who have been to each other's homes, given each other lifts and telephoned each other. Sometimes a therapist's telephone number will be seen as sufficient contact. One group wanted meetings that were less frequent but that included the patient – we provided six-weekly family meetings for these relatives, who had not previously experienced family meetings. If no family sessions have been offered, because a relatives' group was the only facility, then individual sessions can be considered when the group ends.

Summary

Group meetings need structure and control if the necessary work of problem solving and emotional processing is to take place. Therapists must provide a warm, positive atmosphere and be prepared to take active steps to maintain attendance. A range of issues will be discussed, initially practical ones and later more emotional ones.

Part IV

Conclusion

CHAPTER 26

Conclusion

As described in the Introduction, there is strong evidence for the efficacy of working with the families of people with schizophrenia. The problem facing us now is how to disseminate the skills required. The Thorn Initiative was established to tackle this problem and now comprises two national training centres, in London and Manchester. A cascade model of training has been adopted; six satellite training centres are currently operating and a further six are soon to be functional. The successful dissemination of training has revealed another problem: staff who have completed the programme are finding difficulty in putting their new skills into practice. The obstacles here are the attitudes of local managers, the lack of support from colleagues and the difficulty of getting supervision.

The answer seems to be to effect a culture change in the whole organisation responsible for community services (Fadden, 1998). One approach to achieving this is to demonstrate that training community staff in family work is cost-effective. A controlled trial of the Thorn training has shown that trainees are capable of producing the same degree of desired change in high-EE families as the originators of the intervention (Leff et al, 2001). Furthermore, the costs of training and working with families are more than covered by the savings made through reducing institutional care.

An important part of an intervention is for therapists to receive feedback from families. We achieve this by requesting each family member to fill in a Helpful Aspects of Therapy (HAT) form after each session (Appendix 2). This enables therapists to shape their practice in the light of how it is perceived by both relatives and patients. Problems that arise can be picked up early and this should allow action to be taken to prevent therapy being refused.

The written feedback from family members has been encouraging and, as usual, instructive. Below we provide a sample of these comments to give a flavour of what it is like to work with families. Comments on family education and early sessions of therapy were on the whole positive. Trainee therapists were able to instil hope and to set up good working relationships with families.

Effect of education

"Therapists explained the best way to support someone after a breakdown."

"It describes my background." (A patient)

"The discussion I found most helpful was learning why my daughter was feeling stiff sometimes and very weak. I know what to expect."

Effect of family sessions

"Helpful talking about housework, how my wife is going to carry out the task because she doesn't seem to concentrate on quite a lot of things."

"I feel it was helpful inasmuch as I was able to convey my feelings, and circumstances that are happening at this moment, and have been happening for a very long time." (A mother)

"Monitor reasons that may or may not account for my drinking and future support." (A patient)

"My own assertiveness. Trying to see both sides, which is more healthy. Being more flexible." (A patient)

"Finding out what upset my son the most, which is a great help to me."

"At the end of the meeting, my son [patient] apologised for being rude earlier and therefore was aware of the need to be nice again."

"Helpful hints for my own social activities." (A relative)

"Opening up my mother's emotional blackmail." (A patient)

With the HAT form, therapists are able to obtain regular feedback from families on how they thought therapy was going. We found comments on unhelpful aspects of therapy just as important as comments on helpful ones. Therapists can then deal early with any confusion, unmet expectations or dissatisfaction with therapy. Examples of comments are:

"I think this meeting is very important. We talked about my going into a hostel. Well, I am confused about that. I think some more care and understanding are needed." (A patient)

"I did not like the part that was uncaring, e.g. the warnings. And all that the way the therapists shouted at me. That wasn't very nice, was it?" (Perception of a patient)

"My son [patient] seems content to go along as at present and his positive thinking has not so far led to any positive action."

"My daughter [patient] does not want to discuss her problems in front of her sisters because she did not come out of school with 'O'levels, feeling inferior."

"I feel perhaps more could have been achieved if I had been alone." (An emotionally overinvolved parent)

Sometimes what happened in sessions can be construed in very different ways by different family members. Such comments are extremely informative for therapists. The following are some examples.

After an early session with a family

"Meeting was not such a good idea because my sister seemed nervous knowing we are discussing her. It is an invasion of family privacy even though the meeting helps the doctors." (One sister)

"I think it was a good idea that the whole family were meeting and discussing our sister's illness in the comfort of our own home. For the first time I realised that I didn't really know what she was suffering from, but it's now much clearer to me. Beforehand the word 'schizophrenia' meant something totally different to me." (Another sister)

"Other sisters think she [the patient] is lazy. Perhaps it is a good idea to have only me in the meeting." (The mother)

After a session in which the importance of the carers' opportunity to take a break and care for themselves was discussed

"The suggestion of going out to provide a break for myself and my parents is unhelpful." (The patient)

"Therapists suggested that I have a weekend off or away from home, which I agree with. I hope my son will help his self-cooking and cleaning up after him."

Bibliography

Ball, R. A., Moore, E. & Kuipers, L. (1992) Expressed emotion in community care staff. Social Psychiatry and Psychiatric Epidemiology, 27, 35–39.

Bebbington, P. & Kuipers, L. (1994) The predictive utility of expressed emotion in schizophrenia: an aggregate analysis. Psychological Medicine, 21, 707–718.

Birchwood, M., Smith, J., Cochrane, R., et al (1990) The development and validation of a new scale of social adjustment for use in family interventions. British Journal of Psychiatry, 157, 853–859.

Brown, G. W. & Rutter, M. (1966) The measurement of family activities and relationships: a methodological study. Human Relations, 19, 241–263.

——, Birley, J. L. T. & Wing, J. K. (1972) Influence of family life on the course of schizophrenic disorders: a replication. British Journal of Psychiatry, 121, 241–258.

Bustillo, J. R., Lauriello, J., Horan, W. P. & Keith, S. J. (2001) The psycho-social treatment of schizophrenia: an update. American Journal of Psychiatry, 158, 163–175.

Butzlaff, R. L. & Hooley, J. M. (1999) Expressed emotion and psychiatric relapse: a meta-analysis. Archive of General Psychiatry, 55, 547–552.

Dixon, L., Adams, C. & Lucksted, A. (2000) Update on family education for schizophrenia. Schizophrenia Bulletin, 26, 5–20.

Fadden, G. (1998) Research update: psychoeducational family interventions. Journal of Family Therapy, 20, 293–309.

Fischmann-Havstad, L. & Marston, A. R. (1984) Weight loss maintenance as an aspect of family emotion and process. British Journal of Clinical Psychology, 23, 265–271.

Fowler, D., Garety, P. & Kuipers, E. (1995) Cognitive Behaviour Therapy for Psychosis: Theory and Practice. Chichester: John Wiley & Sons.

Hooley, J. M., Orley, J. & Teasdale, J. D. (1986) Levels of expressed emotion and relapse in depressed patients. British Journal of Psychiatry, 148, 642–647.

Jenkins, J. H., Karno, M., De La Selva, A., et al. (1986) Expressed emotion in cross-cultural context: familial responses to schizophrenic illness among Mexican Americans. In Treatment of Schizophrenia: Family Assessment and Intervention (eds M. J.Goldstein, I. Hand & K. Hahlweg). Berlin: Springer-Verlag.

Koenigsberg, H. W., Klausner, E., Pelino, D., et al (1993) Expressed emotion and glucose control in insulin-dependent diabetes mellitus. American Journal of Psychiatry, 150, 1114–1115.

Krawiecka, M., Goldberg, D. & Vaughan, M. (1977) A standardised psychiatric assessment scale for rating chronic psychotic patients. Acta Psychiatrica Scandinavica, 55, 299–308.

Kuipers, L. & Bebbington, P. (1990) Working in Partnership: Clinicians and Carers in the Management of Longstanding Mental Illness. London: Heinemann Medical Books (Part 2, pp. 53–151).

Lam, D. H. (1991) Psychosocial family intervention: a review of empirical studies. Psychological Medicine, 21, 423–441.

Leff, J., Kuipers, L., Berkowitz, R., et al (1982) A controlled trial of social intervention in the families of schizophrenic patients. British Journal of Psychiatry, 141, 121–134.

—— & Vaughn, C. (1985) Expressed Emotion in Families: Its Significance for Mental Illness. New York: Guilford.

——, Kuipers, L., Berkowitz, R., et al (1985) A controlled trial of social intervention in the families of schizophrenic patients: two year follow-up. British Journal of Psychiatry, 146, 594–600.

——, Wig, N., Ghosh, A., et al (1987) III. Influence of relatives' expressed emotion on the course of schizophrenia in Chandigarh. British Journal of Psychiatry, 151, 166–173.

——, Berkowitz, R., Shavit, N., et al (1989) A trial of family therapy vs a relatives' group for schizophrenia. British Journal of Psychiatry, 154, 58–66.

——, Berkowitz, R., Shavit, N., et al (1990) A trial of family therapy versus a relatives' group for schizophrenia, two-year follow-up. British Journal of Psychiatry, 157, 571–577.

——, Sharpley, M., Chisholm, D., et al (2001) Training community psychiatric nurses in schizophrenia family work: a study of clinical and economic outcomes for patients and relatives. Journal of Mental Health, 10, 189–197.

MacCarthy, B., Lesage, A., Brewin, C. R., et al (1989) Needs for care among the relatives of long-term users of day care. Psychological Medicine, 19, 725–736.

Miklowitz, D. J., Goldstein, M. J. & Falloon, I. R. H. (1983) Premorbid and symptomatic characteristics of schizophrenics from families with high and low levels of expressed emotion. Journal of Abnormal Psychology, 92, 359–367.

Mino, Y., Kodera, R. & Bebbington, P. (1990) A comparative study of psychiatric services in Japan and England. British Journal of Psychiatry, 157, 416–420.

Moore, E. & Kuipers, L. (1992) Behavioural correlates of EE in staff patient interactions. Social Psychiatry and Psychiatric Epidemiology, 27, 298–303.

Okasha, A., El Akabawi, A. S., Snyder, A. S., et al (1994) Expressed emotion, perceived criticism, and relapse in depression: a replication in an Egyptian community. American Journal of Psychiatry, 151, 1001–1005.

Parker, G. & Hadzi-Pavlovic, D. (1990) Expressed emotion as a predictor of schizophrenic relapse: an analysis of aggregated data. Psychological Medicine, 20, 961–965.

Sensky, T., Stevenson, K., Magrill, L. & Petty, R. (1991) Family expressed emotion in non-psychiatric illness: adaptation of the Camberwell Family Interview to the families of adolescents with diabetes. International Journal of Methods in Psychiatric Research, 1, 39–51.

Snyder, K. S., Wallace, C. I., Moe, K., et al (1992) The relationship of residential care operators' expressed emotion to schizophrenic residents' quality of life, symptoms and residential stability. Hospital and Community Psychiatry, 45, 1141.

Tarrier, N., Barrowclough, C., Vaughn, C., et al (1988) The community management of schizophrenia: a controlled trial of a behavioural intervention with families to reduce relapse. British Journal of Psychiatry, 153, 532–542.

——, Sommerfield, C. & Pilgrim, H. (1999) Relatives' expressed emotion (EE) and PTSD treatment outcome. Psychological Medicine, 29, 801–811.

Vaughn, C. & Leff, J. P. (1976) The influence of family and social factors on the course of psychiatric illness: a comparison of schizophrenic and depressed neurotic patients. British Journal of Psychiatry, 129, 125–137.

——, Snyder, K. S., Jones, S., et al (1984) Family factors in schizophrenic relapse: a California replication of the British research on expressed emotion. Archives of General Psychiatry, 41, 1169–1177.

——, Leff, J. & Sarner, M. (1999) Relatives' expressed emotion and the course of inflammatory bowel disease. Journal of Psychosomatic Research, 47, 461–469.

Willetts, L. E. & Leff, J. (1997) Expressed emotion and schizophrenia: the efficacy of a staff training programme. Journal of Advanced Nursing, 26, 1125–1133.

Information booklet: Schizophrenia – notes for relatives and friends

These notes are an attempt to give you some information about schizophrenia, its effects, causes and treatment. We will try to describe what it is that has happened to your relative and what it is called.

In the past you may have found that your relative is not his* usual self, that he does not talk to you like he used to, that he may prefer to spend time alone or that he sees and hears things which you cannot. You may also have found that if you try to talk to him about it you cannot persuade him that these things are not true.

You have probably asked yourselves, what is the matter with him? Is it serious? What happens now? You may have found out some of the answers already, but you may not know how they apply to a member of your own family. We hope that these notes will help to answer some of these questions.

In addition to the help and advice of your family doctor, community psychiatric nurse, social worker and psychiatrist, you may find it helpful to contact the National Schizophrenia Fellowship.

The things that may have worried you are the signs of a well-recognised illness. We now know quite a lot about it. For example, we know that sometimes the patient can hear and see things which are not there. His thinking can get muddled, so that it is difficult to talk to him and he doesn't always seem to listen to what you say. This can mean that he loses touch with what is really happening around him and then things he says or does can look odd or unusual. Also, his feelings may change; they may become more intense, so that he appears very miserable or very excited, or they may diminish, so that he loses interest or shows less affection.

Patients who have these sorts of experiences suffer from a form of what is called schizophrenia. Schizophrenia is an illness. It affects people in different ways. The difficulty is that the sort of experiences it gives rise to seem completely real to the people suffering from it but are hard to explain.

---

* 'He' and 'his' refer to both genders.

For instance, someone who hears voices may talk back to them because he thinks they are voices of people who are actually there. Someone who seems to be very cold may not be able to be friendly because his feelings have been swamped by the illness. Someone who is very awkward or does not want to do ordinary things like the rest of the family may be like that because the illness has made him completely wrapped up in himself and he does not realise or care that he is upsetting others.

Because the patient cannot usually explain what is happening in his mind, it is not always easy for other people, even those who live with him like yourselves, to realise that many of the odd or upsetting things he does are caused by the illness. It is especially hard because it is a mental and not a physical illness, so there are no outward signs of anything being wrong. For example, it is much easier to understand why someone with rheumatism can't do so much around the house, or perhaps can't get to work, than it is to understand why someone with schizophrenia may not be able to do these things.

Schizophrenia is not a rare illness. One out of every 100 people will probably suffer from it during their lifetime.

It can affect anyone. It is an illness that starts mainly in people in their twenties, when most people are getting married or moving out of the family home. Both men and women can suffer from it, although it tends to start some years earlier in men. Schizophrenia also occurs all over the world – it is not something that affects just people in Britain.

Symptoms

Now we would like to go into more detail about the sort of things that can happen to someone who has schizophrenia. Certain things happen to almost every patient at some stage of the illness.

Disturbances of thinking are very common. You may have noticed that sometimes your relative says things to you which you don't expect or don't understand. It doesn't seem to make sense. Or perhaps he talks a lot but loses the thread of what he is saying. This kind of thing can make communication between you very difficult.

What happens is that the patient has lost his ability to think clearly and to keep his thoughts in order. Thoughts become jumbled, so they don't always make sense. Sometimes it seems as though there are too many thoughts and the patient feels he can get rid of them only by sharing them with someone, so he may talk endlessly although you may find it hard to follow his meaning. On the other hand, he may suddenly stop talking, because his mind seems to be 'blank'. All this can be very frightening and the patient himself can't understand what has happened to his thoughts. When this happens he may spend a lot of time worrying about it and trying to work out what is going on. For instance, he might think that the neighbours are to blame for what is happening, or that you yourselves are being unfriendly towards him. He cannot be persuaded that this is not true however often you tell him or try to argue him out of it. To him, all these things are real and he will be convinced by them. This means that the illness changes his whole world and he loses touch with what is really happening to him.

Tricks of the imagination

Another thing that often happens is that the patient's imagination plays tricks on him. As a result he hears and sometimes see things which are not there. He may hear noises or voices. Sometimes he will understand what he hears; at other times he can make no sense of it at all. He may hear voices talking to him or about him and he may say he knows where they are coming from, for example the wardrobe, the television or from a part of his own head. These voices can say unpleasant things and the patient often talks or shouts back at them, even when other people are present. Occasionally, they may tell the patient to do things, like opening the front door at night or to stay awake. He may sometimes feel that he must obey these voices and this can become very distressing for him.

Schizophrenia can also affect feelings. The patient loses his ability to feel the right emotion at the right time, so that he may laugh about bad news or may cry when everyone else is laughing. You may have noticed that he doesn't seem to care for you as he did before, or to show his love for you in the same way. There may be fewer and fewer times when you can really talk to each other and you may sometimes wonder whether he still feels anything for you at all. He can't help all this, because his usual feelings have been swamped by the illness and he has become very wrapped up in himself. There may be times when he threatens to smash things or to harm someone he is fond of; this is because he is not always in control of how he feels, but is usually quite unaware of the effect this can have on other people. More often, though, he is shy and withdrawn rather than threatening, and may be easily upset, particularly if you become irritated by the things he does.

From time to time he may realise how much he has changed and how different his life has become. This can make him miserable or desperate and say that life is not worth living. Occasionally, he may become very excitable and overactive and say he has no problems at all.

Something else commonly affected by schizophrenia is the amount of energy the patient has and his willingness to do things. What usually happens is that the patient prefers to be by himself. He may sit in his own room for hours on end listening or talking to his voices or pacing up and down. He may hurry through meals, hardly noticing what he eats and then go back to his room. At times he may refuse to eat at all with the family. This happens because he finds he can no longer feel at ease with other people – he feels awkward and unable to do or say the right thing. He may even actively avoid other people's company, whereas before he seemed to enjoy it. Some patients feel that people in the streets stare at them and avoid going out or venture out only when it is dark.

Sleep disturbance, lack of energy

Often, the patient sleeps a lot of the time and may refuse to get up in the mornings. He may be asleep and awake at completely different times from the rest of the family and this can make it very hard for him to keep a job.

A big problem is when he shows little interest in anything and has no idea what to do with himself. His mind may seem to be a complete blank, or he may pester you to do things to keep him occupied. His lack of energy causes him to take a long time over such things as housework or his job. This can be very hard to live with.

Finally, many arguments can arise over his personal cleanliness, again due to his lack of interest and energy. He may neglect to comb his hair, or refuse to bath himself or clean his teeth. He may dress unusually or refuse to change his clothes.

Sometimes, being careless about some things, he becomes unusually fussy about others; he may insist that his room is kept in a certain way, or that you do not disturb his possessions.

These, then, are some of the general ways in which schizophrenia can affect people, but, as we said before, each individual will be affected in a somewhat different way.

Cause and course of the illness

We have mentioned the sorts of things that can happen to someone with schizophrenia. Now we would like to tell you what is known about why the illness appears, the likelihood of further attacks and how it might affect the future.

Inheritance and other factors

We now know that inheritance plays some part in the development of schizophrenia but by no means explains fully why the illness appears in a particular person. Just because schizophrenia occurs in one person in a family, it does not necessarily mean that other family members will develop it. Often there are no other relatives at all who have such attacks. Neither does it mean that a person with schizophrenia should not have children because they will be affected. All we do know is that there is an increased risk of schizophrenia for children with a parent who has schizophrenia: one out of 10 children of a parent with schizophrenia will develop it in later life.

There are other factors which seem to influence the occurrence of schizophrenia. Research work has been done on many of these factors but at present we can hold no single cause responsible for schizophrenia; there seem to be a number of different contributory factors.

We would like to look in detail at one of these causes which may be important for you as members of the same family. A lot has been written about the influence of the family on schizophrenia. We have no evidence that a family's influence on a child can cause schizophrenia. But, once the illness has appeared, the family can play an important part in helping the patient to stay well. Other features help to decide whether the patient will do well, such as his personality. However, we will concentrate mainly on the part played by the family and will discuss this in more detail later.

Stress, change and conflict

Also, we know that the more things a patient has to cope with in his life, the more likely he is to have an attack. Increased stress can affect anyone badly, but people with schizophrenia seem to be particularly sensitive to it. Changes and conflicts in their lives can also bring on further attacks. We will talk about that later as well.

Most people get better

Well then, what happens to someone who has had schizophrenia? It is important to stress that most people will get better with treatment. They will think more clearly and then the 'odd' ideas will go away. Unfortunately, recovery is not always complete, some patients being left with difficulties, but the overall response to treatment is good.

Some people have only one attack of schizophrenia; they recover from this and never have another. Others, luckily only a small number, do not respond to treatment at all. However, most patients, although they recover from the attack, are likely to have other attacks. These may occur within weeks of recovery or may happen years later. During further attacks new kinds of odd behaviour can appear, but often the same pattern will repeat itself.

In between attacks you may notice that your relative is not the same as he was before. For instance, he may continue to take a long time to get things done. He may say very little when with other people. He loses interest in things and may be content to sit all day doing nothing. This can lead to difficulties in getting or keeping a job and patients may remain unemployed for long periods. If the person affected is a homemaker, the family often finds that he cannot manage to do all the housework he used to. Chores remain undone and the house gets neglected. This means that the family has to rally round and do more.

Finally, even when well, your relative may not be as involved in the family as before. He may stay aloof from family events and seem much less affected by them.

These sorts of things are not done to annoy you. They are partly the result of the medication, partly due to the illness itself and partly due to the person's own attempts to avoid becoming upset and ill again.

How treatment helps

You may have noticed that your relative has been given tablets either while at home or while in hospital. These play an important part in the treatment of schizophrenia. They help to stop the voices in the patient's head, they make him less anxious and restless, and they help him to think more clearly. They protect him against stresses coming from his own experiences and his everyday life.

Treatment takes time

If drug treatment is started, the effects cannot always be seen straight away. It may take days or even weeks before he improves. Even so, the tablets have to be taken regularly. They are not like aspirins, which you take just when a headache comes on. Some patients are not given tablets but are put on injections. These have the same effect as tablets but can be given less often. This is because one injection lasts for quite a long time. It is often more convenient for patients to have their drug treatment in this way, but again it is important that they have these injections regularly.

The drugs used to treat schizophrenia have a number of side-effects, like most other medicines. In this case, the commonest effects are on the muscles. Unwanted movements of the lips and tongue can appear. These are not serious and can be dealt with either by reducing the dose of medicine or by giving an antidote in the form of another tablet. However, sufferers are not always aware of these side-effects and if you notice them you should bring them to the attention of the doctor concerned with treatment. Putting on weight is another common side-effect of these medicines.

Once medicine has been found helpful, it has to be taken for a long time, even when the patient feels better. A lot of people find it very hard to stay on their drugs when they feel well, because it seems pointless. Unfortunately, schizophrenia does not usually just go away. Like many of those with diabetes, who have to take a daily injection even when feeling well, people with schizophrenia often have to stay on drugs to prevent further attacks and to remain well.

In the same way that there is no sudden improvement when patients start drug treatment, there is no sudden change if they stop it. When a patient has not taken his tablets or if he has missed his injections, a relapse does not occur immediately. It can take months until symptoms reappear, depending on the amount of changes and conflicts the patient has to cope with.

How you can help

Drug treatment is not the only thing that helps. The atmosphere in the home and the way daily problems are tackled are equally important.

This is because people suffering from schizophrenia are very sensitive to things happening around them. They are much more easily upset than other people by the ups and downs of daily life. Changes in routine can make them feel unsettled and things like moving into a new house or having to face an examination can bring about another attack. When such events can't be avoided it is a good idea to tell the patient of them well in advance, to enable him to prepare himself.

Life with a person with schizophrenia can be extremely difficult. He may behave oddly, talk to himself, spend all day lying in bed and take hours to get things done. This can make you angry and you find you lose your temper. Or you may feel intensely worried and find that you are always wondering where he is and what he will do next. The inevitable questions arise – what happens in the future if things go on like this and how am I going to cope? – and you get anxious and upset.

Dealing with problems

It is not surprising if you find yourself reacting like this. Unfortunately, it is not helpful for the patient and can make things worse. This is because he is easily upset himself, as we have said, and is unable to take being criticised or fussed over.

The best thing for you to do in this situation is, firstly, not to spend so much time with him, so that you don't get on each other's nerves. It is important that the person leads as independent a life as possible. It will help him to gain confidence and to begin to look after himself again. Sometimes the hospital will arrange for him to spend his day at a day centre or help him get a job. Sometimes, if the patient lives with his parents, it is a good idea for him to leave home and live in a hostel. It may be difficult to accept, but the patient actually does better if he lives a life on his own as much as he can. If this is to happen, a great deal of preparation is needed to help the person become independent.

Secondly, if you have to be together a lot of the time, the best thing to do is not to shout or criticise or get too involved. This is the hardest part as it means that you feel you are not caring enough, or that you worry that your relative will think you are not interested in him. However, in the long run it is better for both of you; he will find things easier if you are less involved with him, and you will find you are feeling less strain. It is important that relatives do not allow their own needs for relaxation to be crowded out by the sufferer's needs.

Most families caring for a person with schizophrenia have to solve similar problems. The purpose of these notes is to begin to give you information, to let you know what you can expect and what you can do to help. If you would like to make any comments, the National Schizophrenia Fellowship would be glad to receive them.

Helpful Aspects of Therapy form

Your name:

Date of the meeting:
Today's date:

What do you think was most helpful in today's meeting? It might be something you said or did, or something the therapists said or did. Can you say why it was helpful?

Did anything else of particular importance happen during this meeting? Include anything else which may have been helpful or anything which might have been unhelpful.

Index

Compiled by Caroline Sheard